CLICKSAFETY™
TRAINING. COMPLIANCE. YOUR FUTURE.

Prep Your Way
Workshops | Online Courses | Workbooks

Associate Safety Professional (ASP)	**Certified Instructional Trainer (CIT)**	**Certified Hazardous Materials Manager (CHMM)**
Construction Health and Safety Technician (CHST)	**Certified Industrial Hygienist (CIH)**	**Certified Safety Professional (CSP)**
Occupational Hygiene and Safety Technologist (OHST)	**Safety Management Specialist (SMS)**	**Safety Trained Supervisor (STS)**

Safety Trained Supervisor Construction (STSC)

SPAN™ Exam Prep is the leading certification exam study solution to prepare safety professionals for exams from the Board of Certified Safety Professionals (BCSP). This BCSP exam prep helps professionals achieve important career goals through advancing competencies for safety management excellence. As the leader in BCSP exam preparation since 1992, SPAN offers live workshops, online courses and workbooks. The self-directed study materials are designed for professionals looking to gain critical knowledge, study techniques, and testing strategies to pass certification examinations.

www.spansafety.com

Dedicated to All Safety, Health and Environmental Professionals

Striving to Protect

SPAN™
ExamPrep

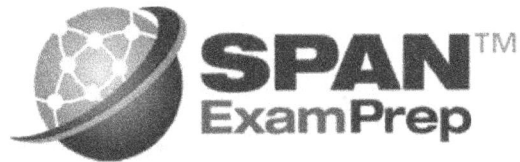

This Publication is not intended to guarantee that the user will pass an exam, become certified an in general may not cover every aspect of the certification process. The information contained in this study workbook is intended to be used in preparation for the Safety Trained Supervisor in Construction (STSC) examination and should not be used as an authority in the professional practice of safety, health, or environmental management.

The Safety Trained Supervisor Construction® (STSC®) Certification are registered trademarks of the Board of Certified Safety Professionals (BCSP).

The opinions expressed herein are those of the authors and no guarantee, warranty, or other representation is made as to the absolute correctness or sufficiency of any information contained in this study workbook.

Daniel J. Snyder, Ed.D, CSP, SMS, CHST, OHST, CET, STS, STSC
Copyright © 2018 by SPAN™ International Training, LLC
402 W. Mt Vernon St #111
Nixa, Missouri 65714
417-724-8348
info@spansafetyworkshops.com
www.spansafety.com

ISBN 978-1-886786-32-5

Contents

Foreword 4

Recommendations for the use of this Study Guide 5

    Safety Trained Supervisor in Construction (STSC) Workshop Lesson
    Plan 7

The STSC Exam and Certification 8

    Eligibility and Examination 9

    Features of the STSC Certification 10

    Benefits of Certification 11

    Description and Analysis STSC Examination 12

    BCSP Certification Matrix 13

    Application and Examination Fees 14

    About the Computer Delivered Examination 15

    Frequently asked Questions about the Computer Exam 16

    Study References for the STSC Exam 18

    The Question/Answer Study Method 19

        Applied Logic: Socratic Method 21

    Example Computer Graphic User Interface 23

Safety Trained Supervisor in Construction (STSC) Examination Blueprint 26

STSC Conceptual Overview 30

    BCSP Code of Ethics 30

    Occupational Health and Safety Management Systems (OHSMS) ... 32

    Management Leadership 36

    Ten Principles of Safety Management 37

    Employee Participation 38

    Hazard Identification and Risk Assessment 39

        Sources for Hazard Identification and Assessment 39

        Hazard Types 40

        Risk Assessment Matrix 43

     Copyright © 2019 SPAN International Training, LLC

Hazard Prevention and Control 44

    Hierarchy of Controls.. 47

Education and Training 48

Program Evaluation and Continuous Improvement 50

Ten OHSMS Strategies 51

STSC Exam Blueprint Competency Quizzes 52

Self-Assessment Quiz 1 Questions...................................... 54

Self-Assessment Quiz 1 Answers.. 60

Self-Assessment Quiz 2 Questions...................................... 68

Self-Assessment Quiz 2 Answers.. 74

Self-Assessment Quiz 3 Questions...................................... 83

Self-Assessment Quiz 3 Answers.. 89

Self-Assessment Quiz 4 Questions...................................... 97

Self-Assessment Quiz 4 Answers.. 103

Self-Assessment Quiz 5 Questions...................................... 109

Self-Assessment Quiz 5 Answers.. 115

Self-Assessment Quiz 6 Questions...................................... 121

Self-Assessment Quiz 6 Answers.. 127

STS Self-Assessment Practice Exam..................................... 135

Self-Assessment Practice Exam Questions 136

Self-Assessment Practice Exam Answers 158

References.. 191

Foreword

This Safety Trained Supervisor in Construction (STSC) examination study workbook was written to help you prepare for the STSC examination. Only BCSP qualified candidates will be allowed to sit for the STSC examination, which indicates that readers using this study guide have relevant experience at the supervisory level.

This study guide is not an attempt at a comprehensive safety management text or supervisory training. Rather the questions and answers presented in this exam prep study guide are representative of questions that may be expected to appear on the STSC examination.

Though the content of this study guide will serve as the main program of study, it is important to realize that additional reading and research may be required to develop an effective study program for an individual to pass the STSC examination.

Achieving the STSC certification is a challenge and can be a professionally rewarding effort that will help you implement health and safety standards in the field and integrate lessons learned into your individual supervisory style.

Integrating adult learning principles applied in facilitated workshops coupled with well-researched self-study methods, this study guide is designed to help candidates pass the exam. STSC workshop and workbook content, concepts and exam preparation techniques have been carefully developed and revised for effectiveness. Nevertheless, significant differences in STSC candidate backgrounds and experiences make it impossible to for the study guide to cover all exam blueprint content in specific detail.

The material delivered in this study workbook has been carefully edited for accuracy; however, if an error is discovered, your feedback would be greatly appreciated. Please send questions and comments to the authors via email to info@spansafety.com

Recommendations for the use of this Study Guide

The STSC workbook is designed by experts in the safety field for use in the fast paced, exam preparatory workshops conducted by SPAN™. Workbooks are also frequently used for guidance during self-study initiatives.

The STSC workbook content is divided into four major practice sessions, totaling 250 targeted questions with detailed explanations. The introduction contains the basic course of instruction given during the STSC exam preparatory workshops, along with the STSC exam information. The text is brief, yet covers a large amount of subject matter. The study sessions are specifically designed to incorporate the STSC exam blueprint competencies and reference materials. These study sessions are designed to allow the candidate at the supervisory level to measure individual progress during the self-study efforts.

Following each practice session are more detailed explanations for correct answers for each practice question. Several study questions offer information about all choices offered as possible answers to enable enhanced learning of the content. Make certain that you study the explanations, don't just memorize the questions and answers.

Reading and focusing on specific explanations will result in greater understanding of exam philosophy. The intensive study process is also a valuable technique for professional development. True learning, comprehension and significant growth occur only when you embrace the concepts presented in the study materials and apply them in the job.

You should review the introductory pages with a focus on the next section on "Study Methods" and then study the materials. Search for a subject or question that gains interest or that is new. It is recommended that you browse quickly through the material to get an idea what you are up against. The practice sessions are designed to be used for self-evaluation and may help candidates gauge exam preparedness. Attempt to take the practice sessions first; then compare to the answer section. These are merely suggestions and each person must use the study techniques that work, based on individual learning style.

The BCSP maintains a reference library of printed material available on subjects contained in the exam blueprint. Suffice it to say that to be successful on the exam, you **must** have a study plan which includes the appropriate budgeted time to master study guide material.

Preferably, you should select a study location that feels comfortable and enables learning without distractions. Schedule enough study time for the STS.

Attending a workshop can significantly reduce study time. This study guide is designed for you to maximize study time, allowing concentration on subject areas known to be on the exam based on the blueprint. By concentrating on the emphasized areas, candidates should be able to maximize time needed for research/study.

The question/answer format is used in the workbooks, with more detailed explanations captured in answer explanation sections. More complex concepts or theories may be abbreviated or paraphrased. This fine-tuning method enables coverage of broad material and serves to expedite learning the main points.

The key is to learn concepts and theories specific to the exam context. The Board of Certified Safety Professionals (BCSP) assumes that all candidates have some hands-on experience in supervisory techniques. Some questions may prove difficult to answer, without actual worker supervision experience and at least 30 hours of safety training.

The study sessions use the question/answer format and are designed for you to become familiar with the style and content of exam questions. Studying of the answer section explanations is highly recommended. The STS examination covers a relatively large amount of general subject matter that is the same on each version of the exam. The STS exam prep study guide has incorporated the specific focus areas on each specialty exam: Construction (STSC) and General Industry (STS)

The Study Guide does not contain the actual exam questions.

Study questions are representative of those candidates may encounter on the official BCSP examination. Candidates must understand the subject area or concept the question is referencing.

Many supervisors prefer to proceed straight through the study guide, studying an area at a time. The results of the initial run through each of the four practice exams will provide guidance in areas that require additional effort. The questions presented are more difficult than those on the actual test, but without thorough study, the exam can be extremely challenging.

Given two hours, you need approximately a 69% or higher score to pass the 100 question STSC examination.

Safety Trained Supervisor in Construction (STSC) Workshop Lesson Plan

Course Description:

The primary purpose of the SPAN™ STSC exam prep workshop is to assist frontline leadership to successfully pass the Board of Certified Safety Professional's (BCSP) STSC exam. This is a fast pace agenda and candidates may require additional study to be successful on the STSC exam. The facilitator is an experienced practitioner and subject matter expert on the exam blueprint domains. Learning strategies include lecture, guided discussion, case studies, self-directed learning, and learner discovery methods.

Orientation/Rules:

- Emergency Exits
- Restrooms
- Breaks
- Silence phones, lap-tops, anything that makes a sound
- We are all adult learners and professionals
- No pictures, audio or video recording
- Ask Questions
- Participate in discussions

Course Objectives:

At the completion of this workshop participants will be able to:

- Describe STSC exam requirements.
- Determine the level of difficulty for the STSC exam.
- Review problems aligned with competencies outlined in the exam blueprint
- Analyze your knowledge gap
- Locate reference materials to enhance knowledge
- Establish a study plan

The STSC Exam and Certification

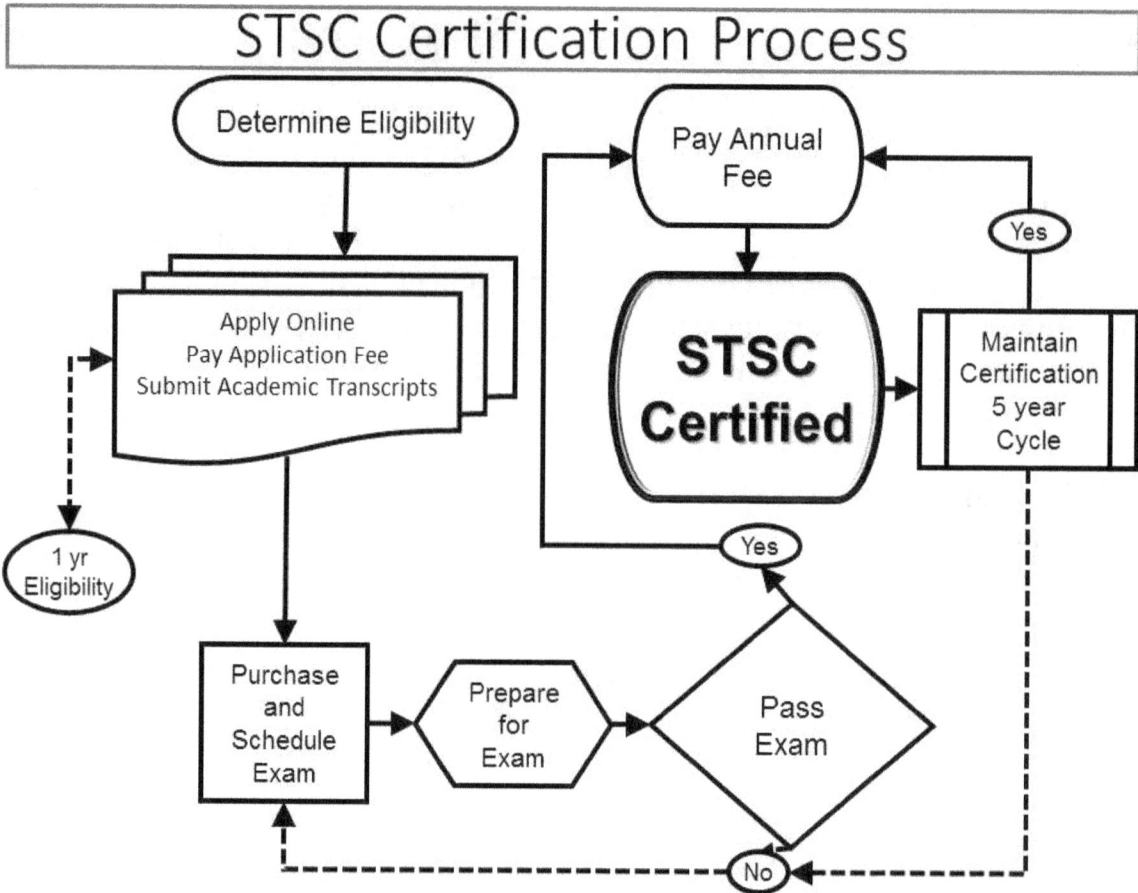

STSC Certification Process

```
Determine Eligibility
        |
        v
Apply Online
Pay Application Fee
Submit Academic Transcripts ----> 1 yr Eligibility
        |
        v
Purchase and Schedule Exam ----> Prepare for Exam ----> Pass Exam
                                                           |  Yes ----> STSC Certified
                                                           |  No
Pay Annual Fee ----> STSC Certified ----> Maintain Certification 5 year Cycle ----Yes--> Pay Annual Fee
                                                           No
```

The Safety Trained Supervisor in Construction® (STSC®) certification is copyrighted and administered by the Board of Certified Safety Professionals (BCSP).

The STSC certification program is intended for individuals who:

1).   Are managers at all levels
2).   Are first line supervisors of work groups or organization units
3).   Have a safety responsibility for a work group that is part of other work duties

Typical candidates have a safety responsibility that is adjunct, collateral or additional to their job duties. Their main job duties are in a craft or trade, in leadership, supervision or management, or in a technical specialty.

The typical certified STSC helps an employer implement safety programs at the worker level through supervisory, safety committee or similar safety and health leadership roles. Safety tasks often include monitoring for job hazards, helping ensure regulatory compliance, training employees in safety practices, performing safety recordkeeping tasks, coordinating corrections for safety problems within or among work groups, and communicating with safety specialists or management.

The STSC safety responsibility is a part-time responsibility, generally consisting of less than 1/3 of the total job duties. If safety responsibilities involve a greater portion of job duties, the role is more likely to be that of a safety technician/technologist or safety professional.

The STSC certification establishes a minimum competency in general safety practices. To achieve the certification, candidates must meet minimum safety training and work experience, as well as demonstrate knowledge of safety fundamentals and standards by examination. Those holding the STSC certification must renew it annually, along with meeting recertification requirements every five years.

Supervisors, managers, safety committee members, foremen, crew chiefs, and other work group leaders play very important roles in making work safe. Safe work practices add to productivity and profit.

Eligibility and Examination

To be eligible for a STSC examination, candidates must possess good moral character and meet the following requirements:

- All individuals applying for the STSC must have completed 30 hours of formal safety and health training through a single course or multiple training courses. Appropriate training includes any safety and health courses, conferences or internal company training, to name a few
- Safety Trained Supervisor Construction: STSC candidates must have two (2) years supervisory experience or four (4) years' work experience related to construction (work experience must be a minimum part-time [18 hrs./week] to qualify).

To achieve the STSC certification, you must pass a Safety Trained Supervisor Construction examination and pay your annual fees.

STSC examinations are offered by computer at Pearson VUE testing center locations around the world on every business day. The examination contains 100 multiple-choice questions and candidates have two hours to complete it.

Please refer to the *Complete Guide* to the *STSC* from the BCSP for eligibility details, application instructions, examination blueprints, and information on testing centers (BCSP, 2016).

Features of the STSC Certification

BCSP examination blueprints are based on surveys of what safety practitioners do in practice. The STSC examination is required for candidates to demonstrate knowledge of safety practice at the supervisory level.

- A simple application and examination process
- Convenient testing every business day at testing centers located throughout North America
- Computer-based testing with immediate pass-fail results
- Distinctive wallet card and certificate
- A national database of STSC certificate bearers available to employers
- A recertification program that helps ensures certificate bearers are current in safety and health matters
- There are two practice areas with the Safety Trained Supervisor Program: STS-Construction (STSC) and STS for general industry (STS).

Safety Trained Supervisor (STS)

The STS® program, which began in 2004, expands the original Safety Trained Supervisor concept to a wide range of businesses and industries. The STS examination emphasizes general safety considerations applicable to all industries and relates to OSHA Occupational Safety and Health Standards found in 29 CFR Part 1910. This examination program requires a supervisor to demonstrate his or her understanding of the principles and practices of supervision in the context of safety.

Safety Trained Supervisor Construction (STSC)

The STSC® program, which began in 1995, is intended for managers, first-line construction supervisors, superintendents, foremen, crew chiefs, and craftsmen who have a responsibility to maintain safe conditions and practices on construction job sites. This program typically falls under OSHA Safety and Health Regulations for Construction in 29 CFR Part 1926 and other construction safety practices. This program emphasizes general job site safety within and among work groups. It does not focus on safety knowledge and skills for crafts or trades.

The STS and STSC certifications hold national accreditation. The STSC® and STS® are registered trademarks and the exams are administered by the Board of Certified Safety Professionals (BCSP).

Benefits of Certification

The primary advantage of certification is that it provides a recognized credential in the industry and BCSP designations are the gold standard. The STSC indicates that a health and safety practitioner has achieved a standard level of qualification as judged by an accredited board of certification. These designations are critical for establishing credibility within the field of Environment, Safety and Health. As the Health and Safety profession embraces the STSC certification, career opportunities will expand for supervisors that have achieved certification.

The demand has increased for field safety coordinators and industrial hygiene technicians tasked with monitoring and safety-related duties at the front line supervisory level. This places the STSC as a unique "stand-alone" certification that provides increased status for Health and Safety Practitioners.

Overall benefits of the STSC certification program for Employers and Owners may include any of the following:

- Thorough evaluation of its employees' fundamental safety knowledge
- Demonstrated competency of its employees by examination
- Increased safety awareness among employees
- Improved safety culture
- Reduced workers' compensation claims and reduced insurance premiums
- Reduced need for safety professionals on smaller projects or assignments
- Improved productivity from better communication among and higher confidence within work groups
- Higher profits from safe work
- Recognition by having employees who hold a nationally accredited credential

Benefits for Employees:

- Demonstrated knowledge of fundamental safety practices
- Opportunities for increased job responsibilities or employment
- Increased value to employers
- Recognition for safety leadership from employers or other employees
- Increased confidence when dealing with safety and health matters
- Recognition from earning a nationally-recognized and accredited credential

Description and Analysis STSC Examination

Each STSC certification examination is a practitioner level exam in length and level of difficulty. It is computer delivered, consisting of 100 multiple-choice questions. Time management should be a minimal concern on this examination the as two full hours are allotted.

This examination is closed book. A letter will be mailed each candidate from the BCSP in approximately 30 days. Official results of Pass or Fail are provided at the testing center immediately following completion of the exam.

STSC examination blueprint is based on role delineation studies of what first-line supervisors do in practice. The top levels, called tasks, represent major functions performed by supervisors. Each task contains a list of knowledge and/or skills required to carry out each task. The percent of the examination devoted to each task is shown next to the task number.

Approximate minimum passing score for the STS Construction examination is 69%.

According to the BCSP 2015 annual report, there are more than 7500 active Safety Trained Supervisors in general industry and construction. Over 1300 candidates completed the STS Construction examination; 83.2% of the candidates passed.

Each certification examination consists of *100 multiple-choice questions*.

This is a basic technical level examination with many of the questions based on not only "book" knowledge, but also on applications of "book" knowledge.

Two hours are allowed for completion of this computer-delivered examination.

After a candidate has successfully completed the STSC Examination, they are authorized to use the title "Safety Trained Supervisor in Construction" and to use the initials "STSC" after their names.

BCSP Certification Matrix

	CSP	ASP	GSP	SMS	OHST	CHST	STS/STSC	CET
Minimum Education	Bachelor's degree[1] or Associate's degree[2]	Bachelor's degree or Associate's degree	Bachelor's or Master's degree[3]	High School Diploma or GED	High School Diploma or GED	High School Diploma or GED	N/A	High School Diploma or GED
Minimum Training	N/A[4]	N/A	N/A	N/A	N/A	N/A	30 hours of SH&E[5] training	Delivery of 135 hours of training[6]
Minimum Work Experience	4 years of experience[7] And Hold an authorized credential[8]	1 year of experience[9]	No experience required[10]	10 years of safety management related experience[11]	3 years of experience[12]	3 years of construction experience[13]	2 years supervisory experience[14] Or 4 years' work experience	Hold an authorized credential.[15]
Application Fees	$160	$160	N/A	$160	$140	$140	$120	$140
Examination Fees	$350	$350	N/A	$350	$300	$300	$185	$300
Eligibility Extension Fees	$100	$100	N/A	$100	$100	$100	$100	$100
Renewal Fees	$150	$140	$140	$140	$120	$120	$60	$120
Passing Scores	100/175 57%	107/175 61%	N/A	106/175 60.5%	116/175 66.2%	108/175 61.7%	**STS:** 61/87 70.1% **STSC:** 60/87 68.9%	119/175 68%
Recertification *(5-year cycle)*	25 points	25 points	N/A	25 points	20 points	20 points	30 hours of safety and health courses[16]	20 points[17]

---

[1] In any field

[2] In a safety and health or related field

[3] from an ABETASAC or AABI accredited QAP program

[4] Not Applicable

[5] Safety, Health and Environmental

[6] In safety, health and environmental-related areas

[7] Where safety is at least 50%, preventative, professional level with breadth and depth of safety duties

[8] ASP, CIH, CMIOSH, CRSP, GSP, SISO, NEBOSH National or International Diploma in Occupational Health and Safety, Diploma in Industrial Safety from CLI/RLIs of the Government of India

[9] Where safety is at least 50%, preventative, professional level with breadth and depth of safety duties

[10] Must achieve the CSP within eligibility time period once CSP experience requirement is met

[11] A minimum of 35% of the job tasks must be related to management of safety related programs, processes, procedures, personnel, etc.)

[12] At least 35% of primary job duties involve safety and health

[13] At least 35% of primary job duties involve safety and health

[14] Related to the STS industry exam for which candidate is applying (work experience must be a minimum part time [18 hrs./week] to qualify)

[15] ASP, CDGP, CFPS CHMM, CHST, CIH, CMIOSH, CRSP, CSP, OHST, STS, or STSC

[16] Or by retaking the STS/STSC exam or earning the OHST, CHST, ASP or CSP

[17] With 2.8 of these points in attending a training, development or instructional technology class

Application and Examination Fees

The entire process of certification generally takes from one to three months. Application and exam fees[18] associated with the certification process are as follows:

- Initial application fee $120.00
- Examination fee (US and Canada) $185.00
- Examination Extension fee $75.00
- STSC certification fee (annual) $60.00

These fees are paid directly to the BCSP prior to testing.

The BCSP uses Pearson VUE to proctor the STS® and STSC® examinations. Exams are given at several Pearson VUE locations throughout the world and can be scheduled during available business hours. The STSC can be proctored on site by the BCSP.

For more complete and most recent information, please contact the BCSP directly at:

Board of Certified Safety Professionals

8645 Guion Road

Indianapolis, IN 64268

Phone (317) 593-4800

Fax (317) 593-4400

www.bcsp.org

---

[18] BCSP fees may change. Please refer to www.bcsp.org for the most updated fees.

About the Computer Delivered Examination

A major goal of the BCSP is to offer certification examinations with a high degree of validity and reliability to promote a fair assessment of a candidate's competency as a safety and health technician. The change to computer testing offered additional flexibility and convenience for candidates.

Testing on computer is done via Pearson VUE (www.pearsonvue.com). Examinations can be taken every business day at many locations throughout the world. Many locations also have evening and Saturday hours. One great benefit of this improved system is immediate test grading. As soon as candidates finish the computer examination, they receive a pass or fail grade. Later, a more detailed result sheet is sent via mail.

Once a candidate has been approved and considered eligible by the BCSP ($120 application fee) and has paid the examination fee ($185), a test registration is issued.

Candidates may register and pay for their examination online by logging into "My Profile" and selecting "Purchase Exam" from the menu buttons. Candidates will have one-year once their application has been approved to schedule and sit for the examination.

Arrangements are made directly with Pearson VUE through a local office or on-line. Some Pearson VUE centers are busier than others, so early scheduling is highly recommended.

At the Pearson VUE centers, a candidate signs in, presents identifications and is seated at a computer workstation. The center provides a laminated paper and a marker for notes. There is a short orientation and practice program to get acquainted with the examination procedure prior to testing. A small clock in the monitor screen corner keeps track of the remaining time.

When testing is completed, candidates will immediately receive a pass or fail grade.

Pearson VUE Testing Center Locations

For worldwide locations, look at the web site www.pearsonvue.com. For all areas not listed, contact the BCSP for testing information.

Frequently asked Questions about the Computer Exam

NOTE: Remember the best and most current source of information on procedures and policies for the STSC computer test is directly from the BCSP (317) 593-4800. www.bcsp.org

Question   How do the test questions appear on the computer screen? How do I make answer selections? Can I back up, or mark questions so that I can come back to them? Do I need to be a computer whiz to take this test?

Answer   Examination questions appear one at a time and look very similar to questions in the study guide. With a mouse or keys, the candidate selects preferred answers and moves on to the next question. They can also mark questions for **further review** or skip them and come back to them. At the end of the exam, a list appears and shows item numbers, answers selected, and questions marked or skipped. The computer test is very user-friendly; you do **not** have to be computer literate to take this exam.

Question   Can I bring food or drinks allowed in the exam room?

Answer   No. A small locker will be provided for all personal belongings, including snacks, purses, wallets, watches, etc. Individuals taking the test may or may not be allowed access to lockers.

Question   What am I able to take into the testing room?

Answer   ID card(s) are permitted. All else must be placed in your assigned locker.

Question   Exactly what is provided in the testing station?

Answer   One laminated sheet of paper, one marker, the computer monitor, keyboard and mouse are furnished.

Question   Describe what the test station is like?

Answer   Cubicles are generally very pleasant, although this may vary with different Pearson VUE Centers. Cubicles are large with a desktop about 3'× 4' with excellent lighting, minimal noise, and padded chairs. Keyboard and mouse take up all space in front of monitor, so calculations have to be done off to the side. The chairs are on rollers, so movement is easy.

Question   Are any children allowed in the testing room?

Answer   Absolutely not. Testing stations are exclusively for adults.

Question   Are there any other people in the room?

Answer   The number of people in multiple workstations will vary with the time and day. Expect a proctor who has a view of the entire room (via glass window and corner mirrors on the ceiling).

Question   How much math is on the STSC examination?

Answer   None. Minimal math skills are needed on the exam, if any.

Question   Are breaks allowed?

Answer   Yes, limitless breaks are permissible, however, the **test is timed** and candidates must sign out and in each time they elect to take a break. Palm Scan checks are administered with each break as well.

Question   Is any identification needed?

Answer   Candidates must possess one government photo ID with signature. Administrators may also take photographs and a palm scan during sign-in.

Question   Will my BCSP letter with my candidate ID number be necessary?

Answer   Yes, because ID numbers are required for candidates to schedule appointments.

Question   Can the exam be scheduled any time?

Answer   No. Certain times are set aside for professional exams. Book your exam time slot several weeks in advance to secure the preferred time and day.

Question   Will I have enough time to finish the exam?

Answer   As with all timed tests, there is variance in required time for completion. Some candidates will find there was plenty of time to finish the exam, including review time, while other people have **not** finished testing in the allocated time. The time per question (approximately 1 minute) is less than the pace required on the written exam. (100 questions in 120 minutes.) Thus, pacing is very important.

Many find the computer method to be a positive, convenient way to take the exam. The Pearson VUE people are friendly and helpful. The cubicles were quiet and well lit. The chairs were comfortable. There was plenty of table space and the computer was user-friendly and non-threatening. Please contact the author at 1-417-724-8348 or email info@spansafety.com with comments.

Your feedback is greatly appreciated. Good luck on your exam!

Study References for the STSC Exam

A free Complete Guide about the STSC certification is provided by BCSP. In this pamphlet is a list of recommended study materials.

The following references have proven to be the most valuable to supervisors studying for the STSC examination:

1. The Complete Guide to the STSC, Application and Examination information. (2nd Edition) 2016, BCSP Champaign, IL 1-217-359-9263. www.bcsp.org
2. *The BCSP Code of Ethics.* www.bcsp.org
3. *Safety Supervisor's Manual (Ninth edition).* NCS Press. Examinees may order this book from NSC, Itasca, IL. 1-800-621-7615. www.nsc.org
4. *Safety Supervision, 2nd Edition*, Dan Peterson, American Society of Safety Engineers, Des Plaines, IL, 1999. www.asse.org
5. *You've Just Been Made the Supervisor...Now What?*, Onion and O'Toole, National Safety Council, Itasca, IL, 2003. www.nsc.org
6. OSHA 1910 General Industry and 1926 Construction Standards. www.OSHA.gov

A complete list of references for information in this workbook can be found in the reference section.

The SPAN™ STSC examination study workbook was written to optimize study efforts. Correctly identifying the best resources is an important element in developing an effective study plan. Most likely all you need is in this study guide, however, the listed references recommended by authors represent most of information needed to pass the STSC exam.

The Question/Answer Study Method

This section of the study guide is designed to assist with exam preparation. It is designed using the Question & Answer format that allows concentration on unfamiliar areas. Critical to this technique is a well-researched set of representative questions and your ability to take advantage of the guided self-study format.

This study method is designed for practitioners who have been introduced to skills and tasks necessary to supervise projects and responsible for implementing a safety and health management system. As adult learners, most are unfamiliar with the process of standardized exam study; however, people generally enjoy the process of learning. The ability to retain what information is important to pass the exam, and reject what is unimportant, is critical in preparing for the exam.

When the study guide is used correctly, study efforts are optimized and passing the STSC examination is more likely. Most professionals will find that the learning process will provide the skills, knowledge and abilities to integrate safety into their individual management style.

The Question-Answer (Q & A) technique of study is appropriate for the STSC. Most research work has been done by subject matter experts and authors who have actually taken the exam, researched blueprint areas of interest and developed targeted learning outcomes. Identified learning outcomes were then developed into questions and answers with thorough explanations.

Learners are presented with questions sets aligned with level of difficulty presented on the examination when this development process is accomplished correctly. The content and layout mimic the actual test questions, allowing candidates to determine if the current knowledge level is adequate, or if a more in-depth understanding is required.

This Q & A technique aligns with research-based methods of adult learning. Individual learners are responsible for determining knowledge gaps, thus, saving significant time by studying the correct information.

The Q & A method includes these steps:

1. *Read Entire Test Question and Options Carefully!* Using existing knowledge, experience, and test taking strategies, attempt to answer question. Skimming or skipping question words or options will result in missed clues.

2. *Process Check.* Review results of each practice session, and then study provided explanation.

3. *Validate Knowledge.* Was this a known or an unknown concept to me? Did I select the correct answer because I had the knowledge base, by making an educated guess, or simply by random luck?

   Note: This critical step in the Q&A learning process determines if candidates can proceed or need to gain more subject knowledge. In additional, self-analysis includes assessing whether knowledge base on this subject broad is sufficient enough to answer questions of similar difficulty on the subject.

4. *Filter.* Either move on or take notes. If comfortable with knowledge on the subject, then move on to next question. However, if not comfortable, then take notes about information needed. The authors recommend that students write in the study guide margins beside the question.

5. *Enhance deficiencies.* Research and study deficient knowledge areas. After completing a set of questions, writing notes on information to study, a knowledge deficiency study plan can be developed. Then research and study the material necessary to enhance the required knowledge. The authors advise focusing on notes in the study guide and staying on subject. It is very easy to wander onto some other interesting subject and lose sight of the desired learning outcome. Keep the goal in mind to pass the test the first time!

Applied Logic: Socratic Method

Consider this representative question, answer and explanation to illustrate and explain the learning process.

Question:

Which is the most correct statement about the function of an electrical Ground Fault Circuit Interrupter (GFCI)?

      A.)   It is a slow acting device.

      B.)   It interrupts the electric power within 1/40th of a second.

      C.)   It will detect line-to-line faults.

      D.)   It is not designed for personnel protection.

Answer:

The most correct answer is B.

Explanation: A **GFCI** is specifically designed to **protect people** against electric shock from an electrical system, and it monitors the imbalance of current between the ungrounded (hot) and grounded (neutral) conductor of a given circuit. *These devices will operate on a circuit that does not have an equipment-grounding conductor.* Except for small amounts of leak-age, the current returning to the power supply in a typical 2-wire circuit will be equal to the current leaving the power supply. If the difference between the current leaving and returning through the current transformer of the GFCI (leakage) exceeds **5 mA**, the solid-state circuitry opens the switching contacts and de-energizes the circuit. Whenever the amount *going* differs from the amount *returning* by a set trip level the GFCI interrupts the electric power within **1/40th** of a second.

How much will candidates need to know about the subject of GFCIs? If electrical work represents a strong area, a candidate probably has significant knowledge about the GFCI and is comfortable with this question and the general subject. Another possibility is that one is basically knowledgeable on the subject, but could use some more focused descriptors. Another scenario may be that a candidate knows very little about GFCIs, requiring more focus on concept details and application techniques. How far into the topic does a student need to explore? The level of detail in the example question may serve as a representative indicator. Beyond the basics, another key indicator is the repetition of the workbook question. Content frequently appearing with only minor changes in question format indicates that the subject matter is important, and authors anticipate the actual exam will have several questions dealing with that subject.

The Q & A method of studying is a proven method. The basic outline is delivered with questions and students can then determine individual levels of subject knowledge. When additional knowledge is required, they can conduct more research and study to develop the required knowledge or skill. This learning technique has proven to be successful for many different levels of adult learners because **the individual** determines what material to study.

Example Computer Graphic User Interface

		YOUR NAME STSC Exam version	Question: 01 of 100 Time remaining: 120 min

Which is the most correct statement about the function of an electrical Ground Fault Circuit Interrupter (GFCI)?

O A.) It is a slow acting device.

● B.) It interrupts the electric power within 1/40th of a second.

O C.) It will detect line-to-line faults.

O D.) It is not designed for personnel protection.

FURTHER REVIEW		PREVIOUS	NEXT	REVIEW

Exam Review Screen

Question 1	Question 11
Question 2	Question 12
Question 3 Incomplete	Question 13
Question 4	Question 14
Question 5	Question 15 Incomplete
Question 6	Question 16
Question 7	Question 17
Question 8 Incomplete	Question 18
Question 9	Question 19
Question 10 Incomplete	Question 20

Questions are Hyperlinked

Fail safe: Are you sure? Y or N

FURTHER REVIEW	REVIEW INCOMPLETE	REVIEW ALL	END EXAM

The Q & A method of studying is a proven method. The basic outline is delivered with questions and students can then determine individual level of subject knowledge. When additional knowledge is required, they can conduct more research and study to develop the required knowledge or skill. This learning technique has proven to be successful for many different levels of adult learners because **the individual** determines what material to study.

Study Techniques

In establishing a good study regiment, it is important to find a place conducive to studying. A good study area should meet the following criteria:

- The study place should be chosen exclusively for the purpose of studying. Avoid using a garage, workshop, family room or other area that represents recreation or other distractions. Find a location that represents a study island, where study is the **only** activity.

- Selected study area should have good lighting, ventilation, be temperature controlled, comfortable and quiet. A large table or desk with internet access would serve as a good location. The purpose is to dedicate a comfortable, personal space with minimal interruptions.

Securing a good place to study should eliminate as many external distractions as possible. You should consider how to minimize internal distractions. Helpful hints for focusing the mind for studying include the following:

- Set realistic time limits, determining what to study and keeping with a schedule. Studying a subject too long at one time can lead to daydreaming which reduces your effectiveness.

- Avoid allowing personal problems to interfere. Personal factors can distract your studies and result in more frustration. If you have serious personal problems, you should consider dealing with them and rescheduling your STSC test date.

- Minimize dealing with outside details. Having too many obligations and/or responsibilities enables "brain creep". Consider keeping a notebook in the study area and jot down appointments and details of projects as these brainstorms appear. It's impossible to totally prevent these details from surfacing, but by documenting them, it may free the mind to resume studies.

- Being physically and mentally prepared to study is beneficial. Much of the following suggestions are common sense, but probably deserve repeating.

  - Eat a well-balanced diet. Increase protein intake; a proper level of blood sugar enhances studying effectiveness.

  - Get plenty of sleep. Establish and maintain a regular work/rest cycle.

  - Exercise is beneficial for more than just an exam preparation. Consider choosing a form of exercise that you enjoy.

  - Avoid mental fatigue. Allocate down time for breaks. The average supervisor should study for the STS exam for two to four weeks. DO NOT attempt to cram overnight.

The suggestions above should serve students well in their study plan. Individuals must establish a study plan that makes sense and can fit into the work/life cycle. If some of the authors' proposed items make sense, students should incorporate that advice into their preparation. If study prep ideas don't seem sensible, ignore them. **Bottom line: Use what works for you!**

Many learners who are studying for certification exams provide feedback that finding a suitable place and time to study are the greatest challenges.

Best of luck on your study program and the Safety Trained Supervisor in Construction (STSC) examination.

The material delivered in this study guide has been carefully edited for accuracy; however, if an error is discovered, feedback would be greatly appreciated. Please send questions and comments to authors via email info@spansafety.com

Safety Trained Supervisor in Construction (STSC) Examination Blueprint

The STSC6 blueprint is effective as of November 30th, 2016.

BCSP examination blueprints are based on surveys of what safety practitioners do in practice. The STSC examinations are required for candidates to demonstrate knowledge of safety practice at the Supervisory level.

Domain 1: Safety Program Implementation • 21.9%

Knowledge of:
1. Established environmental, safety, and health programs for implementation in the field (e.g., program compliance)
2. Appropriate respiratory protection relevant to the job task and associated hazards
3. Incident investigative processes and documentation (e.g., secure site, gather facts, take photographs)
4. How to conduct a job/task hazard analysis
5. Hazards that need to be escalated and who to contact for determination of appropriate controls
6. Sanitation requirements (e.g., hand-washing facilities, toilets, single-use cups, potable drinking water, trash receptacles)
7. Illumination requirements for job tasks
8. Hot work hazards and associated control methods (e.g., fire watch, permit)

Skill to:
1. Evaluate if workers have required qualifications, training, or certifications for job tasks (e.g., power industrial trucks, aerial work platforms, confined space, lockout/tagout, respiratory protection)
2. Identify and evaluate if a worker is fit for duty (e.g., sick, under influence of controlled substances, fatigued)
3. Identify safe and at-risk workplace behaviors
4. Conduct a safety inspection or audit
5. Correct hazards or risks found in a safety inspection or audit
6. Implement corrective actions based on the outcome of an incident investigation
7. Implement appropriate controls for job site hazards

Domain 2: Hazard Identification and Control • 40.2%

Knowledge of:
1. Electrical hazards and controls
2. Excavation hazards and controls
3. Confined space requirements, hazards, and controls
4. Hazardous energy and control methods (e.g., lockout/tagout, blocking and bleeding of lines)
5. Work zone hazards and controls (e.g., traffic control, limited access zones)
6. Hazards and controls associated with material handling (e.g., site layout for materials, proper stacking and storage, lateral and horizontal movements)
7. Struck by/caught between hazards and controls
8. Rotating moving equipment pinch points hazards and controls
9. How to respond to environmental impacts (e.g., spills, pollutants)
10. Appropriate use, care, maintenance, and limitations of personal protective equipment (PPE)
11. Hazards associated with working at heights (e.g., scaffolding, lifts, ladders, stair towers, leading edge)
12. Fall protection systems, components, and installations
13. Hazards associated with walking/working surfaces
14. Hazards associated with poor housekeeping (e.g., rolling stock, slip hazards, blocked exits, fire exposures, material waste)
15. Hazards associated with hand and power tools (e.g., guarding; powder actuated; use, care, and maintenance of tools)
16. Hazards associated with heavy equipment (e.g., crawlers, bucket loader, back hoe)
17. Hazards associated with cranes (e.g., swing radius, ground conditions, overhead power lines)
18. Hoisting, rigging, and signaling
19. Hierarchy of controls

Skill to:
1. Identify if there are risks or hazards associated with the site layout
2. Identify if personal protective equipment (PPE) is adequate for the job task and hazards

Domain 3: Health Hazards and Basic Industrial Hygiene • 12.6%

Knowledge of:
1. Hazards and controls related to musculoskeletal disorders (e.g., proper lifting techniques, buddy system, elevating material to proper work height)
2. Work conditions that could create thermal stress (e.g., humidity, temperature, PPE, duration of exposure, wind) and control methods (e.g., drinking water, warm up area)
3. Chemical hazards and controls (e.g., Globally Harmonized System)

Skill to:
1. Recognize ergonomic hazards on the worksite (e.g., vibration, repetitive motion)
2. Recognize symptoms associated with thermal stress (e.g., heat stroke, hypothermia)
3. Identify hazards associated with inhalation, absorption, ingestion, and injection on a job task (e.g., silica, asbestos, chemicals, lead, welding fumes, sharps)
4. Identify potential exposure to noisy environments
5. Identify if controls are being implemented correctly (e.g., if hearing protection is being worn correctly)

Domain 4: Emergency Preparedness and Management • 11.5%

Knowledge of:
1. Use, access, and inspections of fire prevention and protection methods (e.g., PASS-pull the pin, aim at base of fire, squeeze handle, and sweep side to side)
2. Potential fire hazards (e.g., sources of ignition)
3. Emergency response plans and drills (e.g., natural disasters, weather, crisis, fire, alarms, evacuation, rescue procedures)
4. Required emergency response equipment for worksite hazards (e.g., eye wash facilities, backboard, rescue skiff, first aid kit)
5. How to respond to medical emergencies (e.g., bloodborne pathogens, first aid, emergency contacts)

Skill to:
1. Identify if correct fire extinguishing methods are in place for worksite hazards

Domain 5: Leadership, Communication, and Training • 13.8%

Knowledge of:
1. Coaching techniques
2. How to influence others to achieve desired outcome
3. Effective communication techniques (e.g., repeat back)
4. Negative and positive reinforcement and motivation techniques (e.g., progressive discipline, recognition for correct behaviors)
5. How language and cultural barriers impact the safety of employees
6. How to limit exposure to hazards from multiple trades working in proximity (e.g., scheduling, communication of safety- related matters)
7. What should be documented (e.g., training attendance, inspections, daily safety briefings)
8. All written documentation being discoverable in a legal case
9. Confidentiality considerations (e.g., trade secrets, personal medical information)
10. BCSP Code of Ethics

Skill to:
1. Recognize when to seek appropriate subject matter expertise for additional guidance

STSC Conceptual Overview

It is essential for you to compare your knowledge against what is contained in the examination blueprint. One way to do this is by using a self-evaluation method. A self-evaluation helps determine how well you know various subjects

This section will focus on conceptual themes and exam philosophies. As you prepare for the exam, consider these guiding principles. Many exam questions reflect these concepts.

The STSC is intended for construction supervisors, managers, superintendents, forepersons, crew chiefs, and craftspeople who have responsibilities to maintain safe conditions and practices on construction job sites. These individuals may not have safety as a primary duty, but their knowledge of safety standards and practices ensure safer worksites.

BCSP Code of Ethics

This code provides standards of ethical conduct to be followed by those applying for and holding the Safety Trained Supervisor certification as they assist in the protection of people through their safety responsibilities.

Certificants' shall, in their professional activities, sustain and advance the integrity, honor, and prestige of the profession by adherence to these standards

---

BCSP Code of Ethics

HOLD paramount the safety and health of people, the protection of the environment and protection of property in the performance of professional duties and exercise their obligation to advise employers, clients, employees, the public, and appropriate authorities of danger and unacceptable risks to people, the environment, or property.
BE honest, fair, and impartial; act with responsibility and integrity. Adhere to high standards of ethical conduct with balanced care for the interests of the public, employers, clients, employees, colleagues and the profession. Avoid all conduct or practice that is likely to discredit the profession or deceive the public.
ISSUE public statements only in an objective and truthful manner and only when founded upon knowledge of the facts and competence in the subject matter
UNDERTAKE assignments only when qualified by education or experience in the specific technical fields involved. Accept responsibility for their continued professional development by acquiring and maintaining competence through continuing education, experience, professional training and keeping current on relevant legal issues.
AVOID deceptive acts that falsify or misrepresent their academic or professional qualifications. Not misrepresent or exaggerate their degree of responsibility in or for the subject matter of prior assignments. Presentations incident to the solicitation of employment shall not misrepresent pertinent facts concerning employers, employees, associates, or past accomplishments with the intent and purpose of enhancing their qualifications and their work.
CONDUCT their professional relations by the highest standards of integrity and avoid compromise of their professional judgment by conflicts of interest. When becoming aware of professional misconduct by a BCSP certificant, take steps to bring that misconduct to the attention of the Board of Certified Safety Professionals.
ACT in a manner free of bias with regard to religion, ethnicity, gender, age, national origin, sexual orientation, or disability.
SEEK opportunities to be of constructive service in civic affairs and work for the advancement of the safety, health and well-being of their community and their profession by sharing their knowledge and skills

Occupational Health and Safety Management Systems (OHSMS)

A management system is a set of interrelated elements used to establish policy and objectives and implement strategies to achieve those objectives. A management system includes organizational structure, planning activities, responsibilities, practices, procedures, processes, and resources. The conventional model for a management framework that follows a logical progression of activities aimed at improving the performance of the organization is the "Plan, Do, Check, Act" or PDCA cycle.

An organization may choose to implement a management system for many reasons, such as enhancing business performance through the following:

- Developing a management structure that is effective and responsive to the organization's needs
- Making operational improvements
- Changing the operational culture
- Marketing opportunities and improving public image
- Improving relationships with regulators
- Enhancing the ability to meet regulatory requirements and reduced costs from penalties
- Providing for greater employee involvement, awareness and commitment to performance, and improving morale
- Complying with a client's requirements

Occupational Health & Safety Management Systems (OHSMS's) consist of six "core elements". Each core element is important and necessary to ensure the success of the overall system. All the elements are interrelated and interdependent. The core elements are:

1). Management Leadership
2). Employee Participation
3). Hazard Identification and Assessment
4). Hazard Prevention and Control
5). Education and Training
6). System Evaluation and Continuous Improvement

A summary of the core elements of an effective occupational health and safety management systems (OHSMS) include:

Management Leadership
• Establish clear safety and health objectives for the OHSMS and operationally define the actions needed to achieve those objectives.
• Designate one or more individuals with overall responsibility for implementing and maintaining the OHSMS.
• Provide sufficient resources to ensure effective OHSMS implementation.
Employee [Worker] Participation
• Consult with employees in developing and implementing the system and involve them in updating and evaluating the OHSMS.
• Include employees in workplace inspections, incident investigations, and solutions.
• Encourage employees to report concerns, such as hazards, injuries, illnesses and near misses.
Hazard Identification and Risk Assessment
• Identify, assess and document workplace hazards with activities such as soliciting input from workers, inspecting the workplace and reviewing available information on hazards and risks.
• Investigate incidents that in involve both injuries and illnesses and near misses to identify hazards that may have caused them. The purpose is prevention.
• Inform employees of the hazards and risks in the workplace.

Hazard Prevention and Control

- Establish and implement a plan to prioritize and control hazards and risks identified in the workplace.

- Provide both interim and permanent controls that reduce the risk of exposure to hazards and protect employees.

- Verify that all control measures are implemented and are effective.

- Discuss the hazard control plan with affected employees.

Education and Training

- Provide education and training to employees in a language and vocabulary they can understand to ensure that they know:
  - Procedures for reporting injuries, illnesses and safety and health concerns.
  - How to recognize hazards.
  - Ways to eliminate, control or reduce hazards.
  - Elements of the program.
  - How to participate in the program.

- Conduct refresher education and training programs periodically.

System Evaluation and Continuous Improvement

- Conduct a periodic review of the safety management system to determine if it has been implemented as designed and is making progress towards achieving its goals.

- Modify the program, as necessary, to correct deficiencies.

- Continuously look for ways to improve the OHSMS.

According to ANSI Z10-2012, an Occupational Health and Safety Management System (OHSMS) is defined as a set of interrelated elements that establish and/or support occupational health and safety policy and objectives. The OHSMS should provide mechanisms to achieve those objectives to continually improve occupational health and safety. The illustration below depicts how the OHSMS requirements can enhance the approach to managing health and safety program activities. The circle in the middle of the diagram shows the OHSMS continuous improvement cycle based on the concept of "Plan-Do-Check-Act."

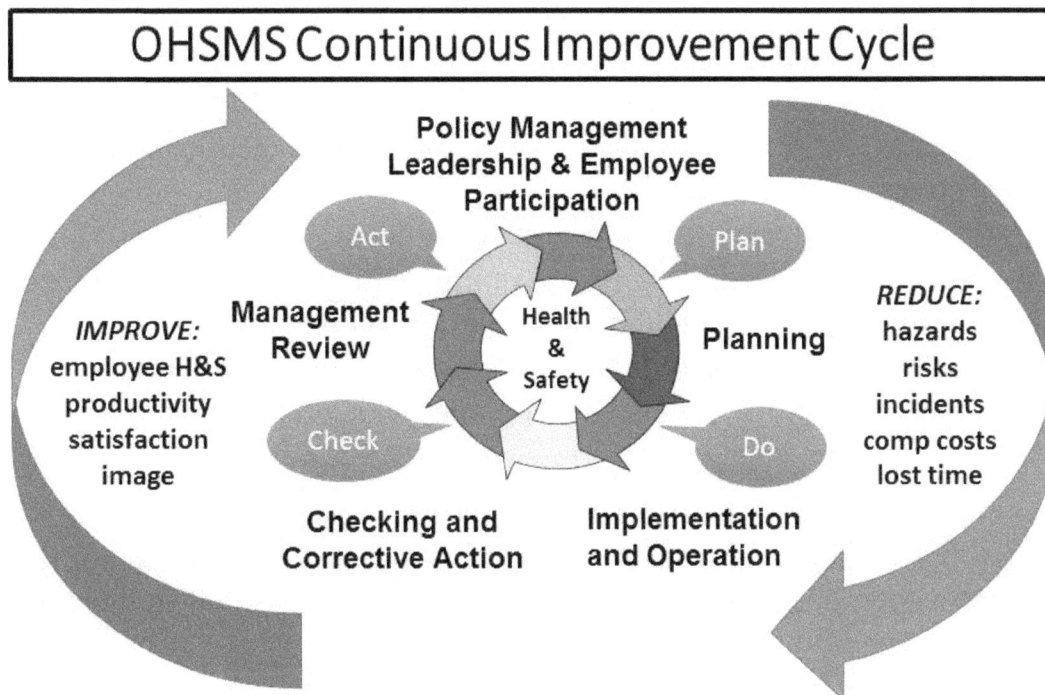

The management system approach is characterized by its emphasis on continual improvement and systematically eliminating the root causes of mishaps. The processes that drive the implementation of the organizational management system facilitates improved teamwork and operational performance. Establish performance objectives, especially for those issues with the greatest opportunity for safety improvement and risk reduction.

OHSMS objectives should meet "SMART" criteria:

- Specific—Clearly defined desired outcome
- Measurable—Concrete metric for success
- Actionable—Written as a concrete action plan
- Realistic—Practical in its scope
- Time-bounded—A specific timeframe is set

Management Leadership

An effective Occupational Safety and Health Management System (OHSMS) requires leadership and commitment from top management. Management leadership provides the motivating force and the resources for organizing and controlling activities within an organization. In an effective OHSMS holds worker safety and health as a fundamental value of the organization. Ideally, this means that concern for every aspect of the safety and health of all workers throughout the job site is demonstrated.

Effective OHSMS leadership:

- Creates safety and health management system policy and procedures.
- Establishes and communicates organizational goals and the pathways (objectives) to achieve goals
- Demonstrates visible management involvement
- Assigns and communicating responsibility, authority and resources to responsible parties and holding those parties accountable.
- Encourages employees to report hazards, symptoms, injuries and illnesses, and identify programs or policies which discourage this reporting.

Successful top managers, superintendents, and supervisors use a variety of techniques that visibly involve them in the safety and health protection of their workers. Managers and supervisors should look for methods that fit their style and workplace conditions.

Examples of visible safety leadership:

- Getting out where you can be seen, informally or through formal inspections.
- Being accessible by incorporating safety and health into operational conversations and standard operating procedures.
- Promptly reward acceptable safety performance and correct at risk situations.
- Leading by example, by knowing and following the rules employees are expected to follow.
- Active involvement by participating in the workplace safety and health solutions.

Ten Principles of Safety Management[19]

1).	An unsafe act, an unsafe condition, and an accident are all symptoms management systems problems.
2).	Circumstances that will produce severe injuries are predictable and can be identified and controlled.
3).	Safety should be managed like any other company function. Management should direct the safety effort by setting achievable goals and by planning, organizing, and controlling to achieve them.
4).	The key to effective line safety performance is management procedures that fix accountability.
5).	The function of safety is to locate and define the operational errors that allow accidents to occur. This function can be carried out in two ways: A) by asking why accidents happen - searching for their root causes B) by asking whether certain known effective controls are being utilized
6).	The causes of unsafe behavior can be identified and classified. Some of the classifications are Overload (the improper matching of a person's capacity with the load); Traps, and the worker's decision to error. Each cause is one which can be controlled.
7).	In most cases, unsafe behavior is normal human behavior; it is the result of normal people reacting to their environment. Management's job is to change the environment that leads to unsafe behavior.
8).	There are three major subsystems that must be dealt with in building an effective safety system: the physical; the managerial; the behavioral
9).	The safety system should fit the culture of the organization.
10).	There is no one right way to achieve safety in an organization; however, for a safety system to be effective, the system must: Force supervisory performance; involve middle management; Have top management visibly showing their commitment; Have employee participation; be flexible; be perceived as positive.

---

[19] Adapted from Dan Peterson, 2003.

Employee Participation

Employee involvement provides the means through which workers develop and express their own commitment to safety and health, for both themselves and their fellow workers.

Employees should be involved because:

- They are the persons most in contact with potential safety and health hazards. They have a vested interest in effective protection systems.
- Group decisions have the advantage of the group's wider range of experience.
- Employees are more likely to support and use programs in which they have input.
- Employees who are encouraged to offer their ideas and whose contributions are taken seriously are more satisfied and productive on the job.

Examples of employee participation include:

Participating on joint labor-management committees and other advisory or specific purpose committees.

- Conducting site inspections.
- Analyzing routine hazards in each step of a job or process, and preparing safe work practices or controls to eliminate or reduce exposure.
- Developing and revising the site safety and health rules.
- Training both current and newly hired employees.
- Providing programs and presentations at safety and health meetings.
- Conducting accident/incident investigations.
- Reporting hazards.
- Fixing hazards within your control.
- Supporting your fellow workers by providing feedback on risks and assisting them in eliminating hazards.
- Participating in accident/incident investigations.
- Performing a pre-use or change analysis for new equipment or processes in order to identify hazards up front before use.

Hazard Identification and Risk Assessment

- Hazard is defined as a condition, set of circumstances or inherent property that can cause injury, illness or death
- Risk is defined as an estimate of the combination of the likelihood of an occurrence of a hazardous event or exposure(s) and the severity of injury or illness that may be caused by the event of exposures.

Sources for Hazard Identification and Assessment

Source	Description
Equipment and machinery manufacturers	Owner and operator manuals typically include (1) warnings of hazards that may be present during operation and instructions, and (2) precautions for safely operating the equipment or machinery.
Chemical manufacturers	Chemical manufacturers are required to provide downstream users with Safety Data Sheets (SDSs). These summarize information about health hazards, and provide instructions on how to safely handle and use the chemical.
Trade associations, insurance carriers, manufacturers, and government agencies	Some trade associations and insurance carriers publish safety and health information. Some manufacturers, and government agencies such as OSHA, the National Institute for Occupational Safety and Health (NIOSH), issue safety and health warnings and hazard alerts directed toward particular products, work practices, or hazards.
Workplace injury and illness information	Data and reports on occupational injuries, illnesses, and fatalities that have occurred in the workplace provide direct evidence of the presence and seriousness of hazards. Most employers are required to maintain logs and summaries of "recordable" occupational injuries and illnesses and to report incidents to OSHA. Incident investigations can uncover previously undetected hazards and ineffective control measures.
Employee safety and health complaints	Employees have first-hand familiarity with the hazards at their workplace. Any prior or recent complaints about safety and health conditions, whether formal or informal, point to potential safety and health hazards.

Source	Description
Medical surveillance activities, and employee exposure data	These results can alert employers to hazards posed by chemical, physical, and biological agents. Use of aggregated results is important to maintain the confidentiality of employee medical information.
Disaster preparedness scenarios	Conducting a "what-if" analysis of possible natural and man-made disasters can help identify hazards that have a low probability of occurrence, but that may have disastrous consequences. Examples include explosions that could be caused by flammable chemicals or combustible dust, hazards that may be created by strong weather phenomena, or incidents related to a criminal or terrorist act.

Hazard Types

Hazard	Source Description and Guidance
Chemical agents	Safety Data Sheets (SDSs) provide a good basis for a developing a list of toxic chemicals in the workplace. When many chemicals are present, hazards of the following types of chemicals should be determined first: chemicals that are (1) volatile; (2) handled or stored in open containers; (3) used in processes where employees are likely to be exposed through inhalation, ingestion, or skin contact; or (4) flammable and stored or used in a manner that poses a fire or explosion hazard.
Biological agents	These include bacteria, viruses, fungi, and other living organisms that can cause acute and chronic infections by entering the body either directly or through breaks in the skin. Sources can include laboratory operations, fermentation processes, or handling of raw food products. They also include exposure to blood or other body fluids or to clients or patients with infectious diseases.
Physical agents	These include excessive levels of ionizing and nonionizing electromagnetic radiation, noise, vibration, illumination, and temperature.

Hazard	Source Description and Guidance
Equipment operation	Ideally, each piece of equipment will be inspected to ensure that all safeguards necessary to protect employees are in place and effective. These include measures to ensure that employees avoid becoming caught in or struck by equipment; burned on hot surfaces; or shocked through contact with energized parts of electric circuits. Important areas of focus for equipment inspection include equipment guarding; the condition of moving parts, parts that support weight, and brakes; and hazards that might arise during maintenance activities
Equipment maintenance	Ideally, the inspection will also include attention to safeguards that ensure that equipment maintenance can be performed safely. This would include such safeguards as deenergizing or otherwise isolating equipment; preventing chemical exposures through appropriate flushing of pumps and other process equipment; releasing stored energy; and use of lockout or tagout to prevent reactivation of equipment during servicing or maintenance.
Fire protection	This part of the inspection would include, for example, making sure that working fire extinguishers are readily available, that flammable liquids and gases are safely handled and stored, and that employees have ready access to emergency exits.
Physical environment	This involves inspecting the facility's walking and working surfaces to identify any trip and fall hazards and ensuring that they are eliminated or controlled.
Work and process flow	The flow of materials and work through an operation can be an important guide to potential hazards. For example, hazards can develop when a product produced at one stage of the process is incompatible with the equipment or practices at the next stage. This could happen in a chemical plant when one piece of equipment produces a hazardous metal catalyst packaged in 55-gallon drums that is then used 5 pounds at a time in another area of the plant. Because of this size difference, employees would need to handle the catalyst manually, causing unnecessary exposures. Producing the catalyst in 5-pound packages would eliminate this hazard.
Work practices	Work practices can be a source of hazards. For example, inappropriate practices for lifting and handling materials can result in back and repetitive motion injuries. When potential hazards are identified, employers can consider whether employees are sufficiently trained to protect themselves. Discussing work practices with employees is particularly important as employees can often identify hazards and solutions based on their day-to-day experience with those practices.

The goal of a risk assessment process is to achieve safe working conditions with an acceptable level of risk. There is no single, absolute definition for acceptable risk and it will vary by organization. In general terms, acceptable risk is risk that has been assessed and controlled to a level that is tolerated by the organization. Obtaining zero risk is nearly impossible as there is always residual risk when operations continue. There are a number of risk assessment techniques and the method depends on the complexity of the situation. Risk assessments may include:

- **Accident/incident investigation**: Although reactive it is another tool for uncovering hazards and management system failures. The primary purpose of the accident/incident investigation is to prevent future occurrences. Therefore, the results of the investigation should be used to initiate corrective action.

- **Brain Storming:** A free flowing group discussion by employees who perform a task to identify hazards, risks, and solutions.

- **Checklist**: Using a checklist is a simple tool to identify hazards, assess risks, and select or evaluate potential controls. Another simple tool is a "What if" method.

- **Job Safety Analysis** (Job Hazard Analysis): A method that can be used to identify, analyze and record the steps involved in performing a specific job; the existing or potential safety and health hazards associated with each step; and the recommended action(s)/procedure(s) that will eliminate or reduce these hazards and the risk of a workplace injury or illness.

- **Trend Analysis:** Worksite Analysis is analysis of injury and illness trends over time, so that patterns with common causes can be identified and prevented. Review of the OSHA injury and illness forms is the most common form of pattern analysis, but other records of hazards can be analyzed for patterns. Examples are inspection records and employee hazard reporting records.

Risk Assessment Matrix

Provides a qualitative method to categorize combinations of indicators and to calculate a risk score.

- Example Risk Assessment Matrix

Likelihood of Occurrence or exposure	Severity and Consequences			
	NEGLIGIBLE: First aid or minor medical treatment	MARGINAL: Minor injury, lost workday	CRITICAL: Disability in excess of 3 months	CATASTROPHIC: Death or permanent total disability
FREQUENT: Likely to occur repeatedly	MEDIUM	SERIOUS	HIGH	HIGH
PROBABLE: Likely to occur several times	MEDIUM	SERIOUS	HIGH	HIGH
OCCASIONAL: Likely to occur sometime	LOW	MEDIUM	SERIOUS	HIGH
REMOTE: Not Likely to Occur	LOW	MEDIUM	MEDIUM	SERIOUS
IMPROBABLE: Very Unlikely to occur	LOW	LOW	LOW	MEDIUM

Risk Level:
LOW: Risk acceptable or tolerable, remedial action discretionary.
MEDIUM: Take remedial action at appropriate time.
SERIOUS: High priority remedial action.
HIGH: Operation not permissible.
Adapted from ASSE/ANSI Z-10 2012. These definitions are provided for illustration purposes and each organization must define these terms as applicable to their process.

Hazard Prevention and Control

Some ways to prevent and control hazards are:

- Regularly and thoroughly maintain equipment
- Ensure that hazard correction procedures are in place
- Ensure that everyone knows how to use and maintain PPE
- Make sure that everyone understands and follows safe work procedures

Ensure that, when needed, there is a medical program tailored to your facility to help prevent workplace hazards and exposures.

Engineering Controls

The best strategy after elimination or substitution is to control the hazard at its source. Engineering controls do this, unlike other controls that generally focus on the employee exposed to the hazard. The basic concept behind engineering controls is that, to the extent feasible, the work environment and the job itself should be designed to eliminate hazards or reduce exposure to hazards.

Engineering controls can be simple in some cases. They are based on the following principles:

- If feasible, design the facility, equipment, or process to remove the hazard or substitute something that is not hazardous.
- If removal is not feasible, enclose the hazard to prevent exposure in normal operations.
- Where complete enclosure is not feasible, establish barriers or local ventilation to reduce exposure to the hazard in normal operations.

Administrative Controls

Administrative controls are measures aimed at reducing employee exposure to hazards. Safe work practices include your company's general workplace rules and other operation-specific rules. These measures may also include additional relief workers, exercise breaks and rotation of workers. These types of controls are normally used in conjunction with other controls that more directly prevent or control exposure to the hazard

Personal Protective Equipment (PPE)

When exposure to hazards cannot be engineered completely out of normal operations or maintenance work, and when safe work practices and other forms of administrative controls cannot provide sufficient additional protection, a supplementary method of control is the use of protective clothing or equipment. This is collectively called personal protective equipment, or PPE. PPE may also be appropriate for controlling hazards while engineering and work practice controls are being installed.

The basic element of any management program for PPE should be an in depth evaluation of the equipment needed to protect against the hazards at the workplace. The evaluation should be used to set a standard operating procedure for personnel, then train employees on the protective limitations of the PPE, and on its proper use and maintenance.

Using PPE requires hazard awareness and training on the part of the user. Employees must be aware that the equipment does not eliminate the hazard. If the equipment fails, exposure will occur. To reduce the possibility of failure, equipment must be properly fitted and maintained in a clean and serviceable condition

Systems to Track Hazard Correction

An essential part of any safety and health system is the correction of hazards that occur despite the overall prevention and control program. For larger sites, documentation is important so that management and employees have a record of the correction.

Many companies use the form that documents the original discovery of a hazard to track its correction. Hazard correction information can be noted on an inspection report next to the hazard description. Employee reports of hazards and reports of accident investigation should provide space for notations about hazard correction.

Frequently, companies will computerize their hazard tracking system which can be as simple as adding a few items to an existing database, such as work order tracking.

Preventive Maintenance Systems

Good preventive maintenance plays a major role in ensuring that hazard controls continue to function effectively. It also keeps new hazards from arising due to equipment malfunction.

Reliable scheduling and documentation of maintenance activity is necessary. The scheduling depends on knowledge of what needs maintenance and how often. The point of preventive maintenance is to get the work done before repairs or replacement is needed. Documentation is not only a good idea, but is a necessity in larger companies. Certain OSHA standards also require that preventive maintenance be done. For example, a preventive maintenance program is required for overhead and gantry cranes.

Emergency Preparation

During emergencies, hazards appear that normally are not found in the workplace. These may be the result of natural causes (floods, tornadoes, etc.), events caused by humans but beyond control (accidents, terrorist activities, etc.), or within a firm's own systems due to unforeseen circumstances or events.

An OHSMS must take into account possible emergencies and plan the best way to control or prevent the hazards they present. Some of the steps in emergency planning include:

- Survey of possible emergencies;
- Conduct a hazarded vulnerability assessment;
- Planning actions to reduce impact on the workplace;
- Employee information and training;
- Emergency drills as needed.

Medical Programs

A company's medical program is an important part of the safety and health management system. It can deliver services that prevent hazards that can cause illness and injury, recognize and treat illness and injury, and limit the severity of work-related injury and illness. The size and complexity of a medical program will depend on many factors, including the:

- Type of processes and materials and the related hazards,
- Type of facilities,
- Number of workers,
- Characteristics of the workforce, and
- Location of each operation and its proximity to a health care facility.

Medical programs consist of everything from a basic first aid and CPR response for sophisticated approaches for the diagnosis and resolution of ergonomic problems. Depending on the size of the site, this may be in-house or through arrangements made with a local medical clinic. Whatever the type of medical program, it is important to use medical specialists with occupational health training.

Hierarchy of Controls

The hierarchy provides a systematic way to determine the most effective feasible method to reduce risk associated with a hazard. When controlling the hazard, first consider methods to eliminate the hazard. This is best accomplished in the concept and design phase of a project.

More Effective

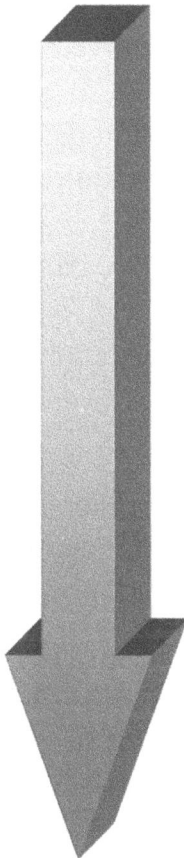

CONTROLS	EXAMPLES
1). Elimination	Design to eliminate hazards: falls, hazardous materials, confined spaces, materials handling, noise, manual handling, etc
2). Substitution	Substitute for less hazardous materials and equipment, reduce energy, etc.
3). Engineering Controls	Incorporate safety trough design such as: Ventilation systems, enclosures, guarding, interlocks, lift tables, conveyors, etc.
4). Warnings	Strategically place signs, alarms, enunciators, labels, etc.
5). Administrative Controls	Standard Operating Procedures (SOPs) such as: Conduct JSAs, job rotation, inspections, training, mentoring, etc.
6). Personal Protective Equipment	PPE assessments may result in the use of: safety glasses, goggles, face shields, fall protection, protective footwear, gloves, respirators, chemical suits, etc.

Less Effective

Education and Training

Education and training are critical for developing the skills and knowledge of workplace hazards and how employees protect themselves from those hazards. It is important that everyone in the workplace is properly trained. This includes the worker to the supervisors, managers, contractors, and part-time and temporary workers.

Supervisors and managers should be trained to recognize hazards and understand their responsibilities. The organization should establish a process to:

- Define and assess the OHSMS competence needed for employees and contractors
- Ensure through appropriate education, training, or other methods that employees and contractors are aware of applicable OHSM requirements and competent in their responsibilities.
- Ensure effective access to education and training, and remove barriers to participation.
- Ensure training is provided in a language the trainees understand.
- Ensure training is ongoing and timely.
- Ensure trainers are competent to train employees.

Training can help to develop the knowledge and skills needed to understand workplace hazards and safe procedures. It is most effective when integrated into a company's overall training in performance requirements and job practices.

The content of a company's training program and the methods of presentation should reflect the needs and characteristics of the particular workforce. Therefore, identification of needs is an important early step in training design. Involving everyone in this process and in the subsequent teaching can be highly effective.

These principles of training should be followed to maximize effectiveness:

- Training needs assessment, will training solve the issue.
- Measurable learning [performance] objectives.
- Trainees should understand the purpose of the training.
- Information should be organized to maximize effectiveness.
- People learn best when they can immediately practice and apply newly acquired knowledge and skills.
- As trainees practice, they should get feedback.

- People learn in different ways, so effective training will incorporate a variety of training methods.

Some examples of health and safety training needed:

- Orientation training for new hires, site workers and contractors
- JSAs, SOPs, and other hazard recognition training
- Training required by OSHA standards: hazard communication, fall protection, operator, electrical, PPE, etc.
- Hazard identification, control and reporting
- Safety inspections
- Accident investigation training
- Emergency drills

Managers and supervisors should also be included in the training plan. Training for managers should emphasize the importance of their role in visibly supporting the safety and health program and setting a good example. Supervisors should receive training in company policies and procedures, as well as hazard detection and control, accident investigation, handling of emergencies, and how to train and reinforce training. The entire workforce needs periodic refresher training to reinforce OHSMS goals and objectives.

Plan to evaluate the training program when initially designing the training. If the evaluation is done right, it can identify your program's strengths and weaknesses, and provide a basis for future program changes.

Keeping training records will help ensure that everyone who should get training does. Training documentation may include:

- The targeted audience and learning objective(s)
- Sources used to develop training materials
- Training evaluation methods
- The date location and duration of the training
- Name and description of the course
- Names of trainers delivering the training
- The delivery materials used
- The trainees participating in the training
- The trainees successful completion of the training
- Certification of training and testing

Program Evaluation and Continuous Improvement

OHSMS evaluation and improvement involves continuous analysis of management leadership and employee involvement, hazard prevention and control, training and education. This may involve periodic review of program operations to evaluate success in meeting the goal and objectives. A comprehensive program audit is needed to evaluate the safety and health management means, methods, and processes, to ensure they are protecting against worksite hazards. The audit determines whether the policies and procedures are implemented as planned and whether they have met the objectives set for the program. This allows for the identification of opportunities for improvement and can inform the strategic planning process.

The success of an OHSMS requires a strategic map that describes major processes and milestones that need to be implemented and maintained to achieve a safe and healthful workplace. This strategy is intended focus on the process rather than on individual tasks. It is common for most sites to focus on the accomplishment of tasks, i.e., to train everyone on a concern or topic or implement a new procedure for incident investigations. Sites that maintain their focus on the larger process are far more successful. They can see the trending issues and thus can make system adjustments as needed. They never lose sight of their intended goals, and tend not to get distracted or allow obstacles to interfere with their mission. The process itself will take care of the task implementation and ensure that the appropriate resources are provided, and priorities are set.

An organization may use a qualitative or a quantitative evaluation system based on its size, operations, services, and culture.

Objectives for measuring safety performance:

- Representative forms and procedures
- Information gathering
- Develop safe work practices
- Appropriate feedback based on data
- Documenting safety efforts
- Justify resources
- Stimulating prevention action
- Reinforcing performance improvement

Ten OHSMS Strategies

1). Define safety responsibilities for all levels of the organization, e.g., safety is a line management function.

2). Develop upstream measures, e.g., number of reports of hazards/suggestions, number of committee projects/successes, etc.

3). Align management and supervisors by establishing a shared vision of safety and health goals and objectives vs. production.

4). Implement a process that holds managers and supervisors accountable for visibly being involved, setting the proper example, and leading a positive safety and health culture.

5). Evaluate effectiveness of recognition and disciplinary systems for safety and health.

6). Ensure the safety committee is functioning appropriately, e.g., membership, responsibilities/functions, authority, meeting management skills.

7). Provide multiple paths for employees to bring forward suggestions, concerns, or problems. One mechanism should use the chain of command and ensure no repercussions. Hold supervisors and middle managers accountable for being responsive.

8). Develop a system that tracks and ensures timeliness in hazard correction. Many sites have been successful in building this in with an already existing work order system.

9). Ensure reporting of injuries, first aid cases, and the near misses. Educate employees about the accident pyramid and importance of reporting minor incidents. Prepare management for an initial increase in incidents and a rise in rates. This will occur if underreporting exists in the organization. It will level off, then decline as the system changes take hold.

10). Evaluate and rebuild the incident investigation system as necessary to ensure that investigations are timely, complete, and effective. They should get to the root causes and avoid blaming workers.

STSC Exam Blueprint Competency Quizzes

- Participate in the development of a site-specific safety plan by detailing hazards and corrective actions to ensure that foreseeable hazards are addressed.

- Establish expectations for compliance with the site-specific safety plan with the contractors, employees and other jobsite personnel using appropriate communication procedures to prevent accidents.

- Verify that job safety analyses adhere to safety standards and in cooperation with contractors, employees and other jobsite personnel to ensure that foreseeable hazards have been identified and addressed.

- Provide technical guidance to jobsite by maintaining a comprehensive knowledge of codes, standards and best practices and informing jobsite personnel of regulatory changes as they develop to maintain a safe and healthful work environment.

- Identify methods for addressing unanticipated hazards (e.g. resulting from change orders, weather, and/or schedule) using professional knowledge and judgment to prevent loss and to modify the site-specific safety plan.

- Activate the emergency response plan when necessary, in accordance with the site-specific safety plan, to protect jobsite personnel and mitigate losses.

- Participate in accident and incident investigations using established procedures to recommend appropriate corrective actions

- Activate the emergency response plan when necessary, in accordance with the site-specific safety plan, to protect jobsite personnel and mitigate losses.

- Participate in accident and incident investigations using established procedures to recommend appropriate corrective actions.

- Perform worksite assessments in accordance with regulations, best practices and the site-specific safety plan using a walkthrough, in order to verify compliance and identify hazards and potential hazards in the work place.

- Recommend corrective actions for hazards and potential hazards identified in worksite assessment using professional knowledge and judgment, in order to prevent loss and ensure compliance with regulations and site-specific safety plan.

- Participate in regulatory safety, health and environmental inspections in accordance with directions provided in the site-specific safety plan, in order to facilitate the inspection process.

- Determine training needs based on job safety analyses, regulatory requirements, trends, and/or observations made in worksite audits to develop appropriate training.

- Deliver training that addresses required program elements using program management guidelines, on-the-job training and evaluation and formal and informal resources to deliver appropriate training.

- Conduct site-specific job safety orientation and training using appropriate instructional methods to address jobsite hazards and abatement procedures, as identified in the job safety analyses.

- Participate in jobsite safety meetings with all crafts by leading discussions, demonstrating safe practices, etc. to inform jobsite personnel of potential risks.

- Maintain complete and accurate records in all aspects of safety program in accordance with established protocol to document interventions, losses and audit findings and to support future decision making.

- Maintain ongoing competence by participating in the Certification Maintenance program to ensure currency and adhere to best practices.

- Adhere to ethical standards for behavior in accordance with the STS Code of Professional Conduct to protect interests of the stakeholders.

Self-Assessment Quiz 1 Questions

1). When in use, electrical power tools and cords must:

   A) Make use of ground fault circuit interrupters.
   B) Be a two wire, double insulated construction.
   C) Be grounded to operate properly.
   D) Make use of ground fault circuit interrupters or be part of an assured equipment grounding conductor program.

2). If a supervisor is given authority by the General Manager to stop operations site whenever he or she observes an imminent danger situation, which of the following correctly identifies that authority?

   A) Staff authority.
   B) Staff to line authority.
   C) Authority of delegation.
   D) Functional authority.

3). As a certified Safety Trained Supervisor, you are expected to

   A) Ensure the profitability of company as your first priority.
   B) Seek methods to improve personal knowledge and understanding of methods, techniques and practices for workers' protection.
   C) Seek to improve personal knowledge of financial and accounting practices related to supervising industrial activities.
   D) Carefully assess situation and problems to identify the most productive methods of completing construction tasks, while working to maintain work area in a manner that will pass regulatory inspection.

4). Arrange the following hazard control steps in the most appropriate sequence: (1) guard hazard (2) engineer out hazard, if possible (3) educate personnel.

   A) 2,1,3
   B) 3,1,2
   C) 1,2,3
   D) 3,2,1

5). Which action is preferred when dealing with minor infractions of work safety rules?

        A) Oral reprimand.
        B) Written reprimand.
        C) No response or consequence.
        D) Suspension.

6). System safety analysis can be applied to which of the following?

        A) Generally, only on most complex of processes or systems.
        B) Very simple systems with only a single component.
        C) Any system that has interacting components.
        D) Any system, only after some loss has occurred.

7). What should a supervisor do when a crew must walk across an area with open floor holes to get to their work area?

        A) Warn them of hazards and tell them to avoid the holes.
        B) Let them walk through.
        C) Have floor holes covered before allowing workers to walk across.
        D) Have the floor holes covered and inform crew of load surface restrictions.

8). The strongest motivator, according to the contemporary motivation theory is:

        A) Fear of upper management.
        B) Status among peers.
        C) Recognition of achievement for performance.
        D) Pay as compared to peers.

9). Management has increased work hours and is pushing for more productivity. As STS, you are concerned about some of the safety risks associated with this production schedule. You should:

        A) Report concern to the US Department of Labor (DOL).
        B) Tell workers to launch a work slowdown.
        C) Inform/communicate increased hazards due to increased production and verify that risk is acceptable.
        D) Do not challenge the management; accept the production schedule.

10). The best evaluation of tasks descriptor involving steps, hazards and solutions is?

    A) System Safety Analysis (SSA).
    B) Fault Tree Analysis (FTA).
    C) Job Safety Analysis (JSA).
    D) Management Oversight and Risk Tree (MORT).

11). What minimum PPE is required for a worker in a grinding operation?

    A) None, there is not a hazard.
    B) Eye and face protection.
    C) Hearing, eye, head and foot protection.
    D) Hearing, eye, head, foot and respiratory protection.

12). **Minimally,** ___ authorized attendant(s) shall be on duty outside of the space during permit required confined space operations and shall be responsible for securing immediate aid, keeping an accurate count of entrants in case of emergency.

    A) Zero.
    B) One.
    C) Two.
    D) Three.

13). A medical questionnaire required when safety workers place an employee in respiratory protection must be evaluated by whom?

    A) The industrial hygienist.
    B) The safety director.
    C) A licensed health care professional.
    D) Any supervisor in the employee's chain.

14). In construction, each employee on a walking/working surface (horizontal and vertical surface) with an unprotected side or edge which is ___ feet or more above a lower level shall be protected from falling by the use of guardrail systems, safety net systems, or personal fall arrest systems.

    A) 3
    B) 6
    C) 10
    D) 4

15). A crew member deliberately violates a safety procedure. What should be done?

     A) Do nothing.
     B) Stop work, write formal complaint and explain.
     C) Talk with worker to explain what he/she was doing was wrong, and allow him/her to return to work.
     D) Summon the Safety Supervisor.

16). Each employee on a scaffold more than _____ feet above a lower level shall be provided with fall protection to prevent from falling to that lower level.

     A) 3
     B) 6
     C) 10
     D) 12

17). Professional ethics refers to:

     A) A set of principles and standards that guide the actions of professionals that are often referenced in civil or criminal cases involving professional conduct.
     B) The laws that the professional must comply with or face possible civil and criminal charges.
     C) A set of bylaws established to assure the members of an organization must follow.
     D) Voluntary rules expected of members of professional associations.

18). When working on scaffold 20 feet high, who must approve the scaffold for use?

     A) The Superintendent.
     B) The Supervisor.
     C) The Competent Person.
     D) The Engineer.

19). What mishaps require reporting to OSHA within 8 hours?

    A) The first aid injury of an employee that required hospitalization, because of a work-related incident.

    B) The fatality of one or more employees, because of a work-related incident.

    C) The injury of more than three employees that requires hospitalization or involves traumatic amputation or broken bones, because of a work-related incident.

    D) The transport of five or more workers to a hospital, because of a work-related incident.

20). A guardrail system's **MAJOR** components include?

    A) Top rails, mid rails, screens, nets.

    B) Top rails, toe boards, anchor points.

    C) Top rails, toe boards, screens, anchor points.

    D) Top rails, mid rails, toe boards, screens.

21). Incident investigations are conducted **PRIMARILY** to:

    A) Discipline rule violators.

    B) Provide regulatory agencies information.

    C) Satisfy the insurance carrier.

    D) Determine causal conditions and prevent future mishaps.

22). Accident analysis is **PRIMARILY** used as a(n)?

    A) Performance review system.

    B) Federal agency reporting system.

    C) Baseline for goals.

    D) Indicator of problem areas.

23). For injury accident analysis, information sources include all the following **EXCEPT**?

    A) First-aid report.

    B) Insurance rate table.

    C) First Report of Injury form.

    D) Supervisor accident investigation.

24). The **MAJOR** cause of serious industrial injuries is?

    A) Slips, trips and falls.
    B) Lack of PPE (Personal Protective Equipment).
    C) Struck by falling objects.
    D) Electrical shocks.

25). If a worker is injured while performing duties assigned by the employer, the injury is considered:

    A) Non-work related.
    B) Work related.
    C) Non-compensable.
    D) Employee misconduct.

Self-Assessment Quiz 1 Answers

1)   Answer D.

Electrical power tools and cords used in construction must make use of ground fault circuit interrupters or an assured equipment grounding conductor program. An assured equipment grounding conductor program requires extensive work site controls, inspections and recordkeeping.

2)   Answer D.

The operational control delegated the safety supervisor to shut down dangerous jobs by the General Manager is functional or line authority. This authority, or lack of it, is hotly debated by safety and health professionals.   The General Managers need to reserve strength over line managers because of conflicts between organizational demands and safety concerns. The act of delegation of authority is, in and of itself, a strong commitment by senior management to the safety process.

3)   Answer B.

Seek methods to improve your knowledge and understanding of methods, techniques and practices for protection of workers. STS Code of Ethics

4)   Answer A.

Engineering is always the first and most successful method of dealing with a problem. The second choice is to guard the hazard, and finally to educate the human element.

5)   Answer A.

Progressive companies believe the proper way to deal with minor rule infractions is to issue an oral reprimand for the first offense. Progressive discipline is then administered for additional violations.

6)   Answer C.

The discipline of system safety can be applied to almost any system that has interacting components. It is an application of systematic and forward-looking techniques to identify and control hazards. Discipline is most effective if it begins within the conceptual phases of project development and should continue throughout the entire life of the project or product.

7)   Answer D.

Have the floor holes covered and inform your crew of the load surface restrictions.

8)   Answer C.

Current theory holds that recognition of achievement is the single most important motivator.

9)   Answer C.

Informing/communicating to upper management the increased hazards due to increased production and verifying that risk is acceptable is the best solution.

10)   Answer C.

Job Safety Analysis is a systematic analysis of job elements. It results in an in-depth evaluation by workers and first line supervisors of individual steps and hazards. JSAs also offer protective measures or solutions to identified hazards.

Option "A" (System Safety Analysis) is a broad term covering all of the various system safety tools used in analysis of system risk.

Option "B", Fault Tree Analysis is the process of using deductive logic to determine the combination of events that caused a hazardous event to occur. It normally is accompanied by a companion report that evaluates the overall likelihood of failure and provides solutions to findings discovered in FTA.

Option "D" MORT, Management Oversight and Risk Tree is a formal decision tree used in evaluation of safety programs or as an accident investigation tool. The tool is exhaustive, offering about 1500 events to be evaluated. For this reason, it is often considered overkill for all but the largest evaluations or mishaps. However, the system logic is sound and recently several practitioners have produced mini-mort charts that have proven to be useful tools for smaller applications.

11)   Answer B.

Without further information of the actual work conditions, the likely minimum required PPE would be eye, face. (OSHA) Protective equipment, including personal protective equipment for eyes, face, head, and extremities, protective clothing, respiratory devices, and protective shields and barriers, shall be provided, used, and maintained in a sanitary and reliable condition wherever necessary by reason of hazards of processes or environment, chemical hazards, radiological hazards, or mechanical irritants encountered in a manner capable of causing injury or impairment in function of any body part through absorption, inhalation or physical contact.

12)   Answer B.

A confined space has limited openings for entry or exit, is large enough for entering and working, and is not designed for continuous worker occupancy. Confined spaces include underground vaults, tanks, storage bins, manholes, pits, silos, underground utility vaults and pipelines. See 29 CFR 1910.146.

Permit-required confined spaces are confined spaces that:

- May contain a hazardous or potentially hazardous atmosphere.
- May contain a material which can engulf an entrant.
- May contain walls that converge inward or floors that slope downward and taper into a smaller area which could trap or asphyxiate an entrant.
- May contain other serious physical hazards such as unguarded machines or exposed live wires.
- Must be identified by the employer who must inform exposed employees of the existence and location of such spaces and their hazards.

Entrants maintain contact at all times with a trained attendant either visually, via phone, or by two-way radio. This monitoring system enables the attendant and entry supervisor to order entrants to evacuate and to alert appropriately trained rescue personnel to rescue entrants when needed.
The employer must ensure that at least one attendant is stationed outside the permit space for the duration of entry operations.

The attendant is required to:

- Remain outside the permit space during entry operations unless relieved by another authorized attendant;
- Perform non-entry rescues when specified by the employer's rescue procedure;
- Know existing and potential hazards, including information on the mode of exposure, signs or symptoms, consequences and physiological effects;
- Maintain communication with and keep an accurate account of those workers entering the permit space;
- Order evacuation of the permit space when:
- A prohibited condition exists;
- A worker shows signs of physiological effects of hazard exposure;
- An emergency outside the confined space exists; and
- The attendant cannot effectively and safely perform required duties.
- Summon rescue and other services during an emergency;
- Ensure that unauthorized people stay away from permit spaces or exit immediately if they have entered the permit space;
- Inform authorized entrants and the entry supervisor if any unauthorized person enters the permit space; and
- Perform no other duties that interfere with the attendant's primary duties

13)   Answer C.

1910.134(e)(2)(i)

The employer shall identify a physician or other licensed health care professional (PLHCP) to perform medical evaluations using a medical questionnaire or an initial medical examination that obtains the same information as the medical questionnaire.

14)   Answer B.

Employers must set up the work place to prevent employees from falling off of overhead platforms, elevated work stations or into holes in the floor and walls. OSHA requires that fall protection be provided at elevations of four feet in general industry workplaces, five feet in shipyards, six feet in the construction industry and eight feet in longshoring operations. In addition, OSHA requires that fall protection be provided when working over dangerous equipment and machinery, regardless of the fall distance.

To prevent employees from being injured from falls, employers must:

- Guard every floor hole into which a worker can accidentally walk (using a railing and toe-board or a floor hole cover).
- Provide a guard rail and toe-board around every elevated open sided platform, floor or runway.
- Regardless of height, if a worker can fall into or onto dangerous machines or equipment (such as a vat of acid or a conveyor belt) employers must provide guardrails and toe-boards to prevent workers from falling and getting injured.
- Other means of fall protection that may be required on certain jobs include safety harness and line, safety nets, stair railings and hand rails.

15) Answer B.

Stop work, write formal disciplinary report, and explain reasoning to worker.. The key to disciplinary reporting in this instance is that the worker deliberately violated the rule.

16) Answer C.

1926.451(g)(1) – Fall Protection

Each employee working on scaffold more than 10 feet (3.1 m) above a lower level shall be protected from falling to that lower level. Paragraphs (g)(1)(i) through (vii) of this section, establish the types of fall protection to be provided to the employees on each type of scaffold. Paragraph (g)(2) of this section addresses fall protection for scaffold erectors and dismantlers.

Note to paragraph (g)(1): The fall protection requirements for employees installing suspension scaffold support systems on floors, roofs, and other elevated surfaces are set forth in subpart M.

Each employee on a boatswains' chair, catenary scaffold, float scaffold, needle beam scaffold, or ladder jack scaffold shall be protected by a personal fall arrest system.

Each employee on a single-point or two-point adjustable suspension scaffold shall be protected by both a personal fall arrest system and guardrail system.

Each employee on a crawling board (chicken ladder) shall be protected by a personal fall arrest system, a guardrail system (with minimum 200-pound top rail capacity), or by a three-fourth inch (1.9 cm) diameter grab-line, or equivalent handhold, securely fastened beside each crawling board.

Each employee on a self-contained adjustable scaffold shall be protected by a guardrail system (with minimum 200-pound top rail capacity) when the platform is supported by the frame structure, and by both a personal fall arrest system and a guardrail system (with minimum 200-pound top rail capacity) when the platform is supported by ropes.

17)   Answer A.

Ethics refers to a set of principles and standards that guide the actions of professionals that are often referenced in civil or criminal cases involving professional conduct. A basic definition of ethics is: moral principles or practice. Professional ethics require consideration of additional areas including, professional values, culture, acceptable standards of behavior and legality. Professionals will likely face ethical dilemmas during their career. Some day-to-day ethical dilemmas are simple to determine the correct course of action; others are not as clear.

18)   Answer C.

1926.451(a)(3) No scaffold shall be erected, moved, dismantled, or altered except under the supervision of competent persons.

1926.451(b)(16) All wood pole scaffolds 60 feet or less in height shall be constructed and erected in accordance with Tables L-4 to 10. If they are over 60 feet in height, they shall be designed by a qualified engineer competent in this field, and it shall be constructed and erected in accordance with such design.

1926.451(c)(4) and (5) Tube and coupler scaffolds shall be limited in heights and working levels to those permitted in Tables L- 10, 11, and 12. Drawings and specifications of all tube and coupler scaffolds above the limitations in Tables L- 10, 11, and 12 shall be designed by a qualified engineer competent in this field. All tube and coupler scaffolds shall be constructed and erected to support four times the maximum intended loads, as set forth in Tables L- 10, 11, and 12, or as set forth in specifications by a licensed professional engineer competent in this field.

1926.451(d)(9) Drawings and specifications for all frame scaffolds over 125 feet in height above base plates shall be designed by a registered professional engineer.

1926.451(g)(3) Unless outrigger scaffolds are designed by a registered professional engineer competent in this field, they shall be constructed and erected in accordance with Table L-13. Outrigger scaffolds, designed by a registered professional engineer, and constructed and erected in accordance with such design.

19)   Answer B.

Employers must report the following events to OSHA:
- All work-related fatalities
- All work-related in-patient hospitalizations of one or more employees
- All work-related amputations
- All work-related losses of an eye

Employers must report work-related fatalities within **8 hours of finding out about it.**

For any in-patient hospitalization, amputation, or eye loss employers must report the incident within 24 hours of learning about it.

Only fatalities occurring within 30 days of the work-related incident must be reported to OSHA. Further, for an inpatient hospitalization, amputation or loss of an eye, then incidents must be reported to OSHA only if they occur within 24 hours of the work-related incident.

- Each report required by this section shall relate the following information:
- Establishment name
- location of incident
- Time of incident
- Number of fatalities or hospitalized employee(s)
- Name(s) of injured employee(s)
- Contact person
- Phone number
- Description of incident

20)   Answer D.

The major components of a guardrail system are top rails, mid rails, toe boards and screens.

21)   Answer D.

Accidents or mishaps are investigated by safety and health professionals to determine root cause factors and to prevent similar future occurrences by implementing appropriate corrective actions. This goal must be kept in mind throughout the investigation process. Many times, other investigations are being conducted for other reasons. For example, security, personnel, or possibly even the legal staff, may be interested in facts surrounding any unusual event. These investigations usually are searching for discipline, reimbursement, protection from liability/litigation or assessment of blame. It is not uncommon for safety professional to be drawn into these investigations because of their investigative skills and in-depth knowledge of the job site. However, it is imperative that accident prevention investigations be separated from discipline investigations if one is to find the true cause factors. Firing the person who had the accident will rarely prevent the next one.

22)   Answer D.

The goal of accident analysis is to uncover problem areas.

23)   Answer B.

The insurance rate table provides little or no useful information for analysis of accidents since it is most often based on experience.

24)   Answer A.

Falls are, by far, the most common cause of serious construction injuries.

25)   Answer B.

When a worker is injured while performing duties assigned by the employer, the injury is considered work-related.

Self-Assessment Quiz 2 Questions

1).   The two general areas of accident costs include:

    A) Budgeted and non-budgeted.
    B) Insured and uninsured.
    C) Direct and indirect.
    D) Direct and uninsured.

2).   **MINOR** incident and near miss investigations are **BEST** conducted by the:

    A) Supervisor.
    B) Manager.
    C) Chief Executive Officer.
    D) Safety Engineer.

3).   The investigation of serious or fatal mishaps should be led by:

    A) A senior management official.
    B) The site safety practitioner.
    C) The supervisor.
    D) The insurance investigator.

4).   Often several accident investigators will be at the scene of an accident at the same time due to varying reasons for gathering information. Which of the following is the **LEAST** important task with respect to the STSC's accident investigation responsibilities?

    A) Arriving first on the scene.
    B) Preventing a second accident.
    C) Preserving as much evidence as possible.
    D) Taking care of, and/or transporting the injured and/or dead.

5). While interviewing witnesses to an accident or participants in the event, investigators often find themselves talking to hostile and very defensive people. Which of the following methods would **MOST LIKELY** result in an honest and truthful statement from these interviewees?

A) Inform these people that all that they say will be written down and filed; thus, telling the truth is imperative.

B) Tell them the information will only be used for accident prevention purposes and no disciplinary actions will result from the investigation.

C) Inform the person that it would be appreciated if they would tell the truth since it may help secure investigator's current position within the company and should not affect them.

D) Tell them that they are supposed to be informed of their rights, but will not be, so they have nothing to fear because anything they say cannot be used against them.

6). Throughout accident investigations, the interviewing of witnesses is often required to determine facts relative to the event. Which of the following choices offers the **BEST** place to conduct interviews for safety investigations?

A) In a secure board room equipped with sound recording devices.

B) Privately in a conference room.

C) At the employees' work area.

D) In your office with door shut.

7). The **BEST** descriptor of the legal premise of "chain of custody" is?

A) Secure storage.

B) Documentation of possession.

C) Ownership.

D) Personal knowledge.

8). When should an accident investigation begin?

A) Within 48 hours of the time the accident scene is secured; that is, after emergency services have left the site.

B) Immediately after the incident, the sooner the better.

C) As soon as possible, realizing that protection of the injured and prevention of a second accident will take precedence.

D) As soon as all legal notifications have been made and the scene has been secured against destruction of evidence.

9). The **PRIMARY** root cause(s) for accidents are:

A) Human factors.

B) Environmental factors.

C) Physical factors.

D) Combinations of causal factors.

10). The action taken to free equipment from any electric connection and/or electric charge is called:

A) De-energize.

B) Safe.

C) Guard.

D) Ground.

11). Collars, couplings, cams, clutches, flywheels, shaft ends, spindles, meshing gears, and horizontal or vertical shafting are all examples of what type of mechanical hazard?

A) Impact hazard.

B) Shearing action.

C) Nip point.

D) Rotating motion.

12). Which of the following descriptions **BEST** fits that of a "Competent Person"?

  A) The person required at confined space, and hoisting & rigging, and excavation & trenching job sites.

  B) The supervisor with the ability to identify existing and future hazards on the job site and who reports directly to the person responsible for operation.

  C) The person who has authority to shut down the operation anytime the risk analysis indicates that a moderate or greater hazard is reasonably expected to cause injury to workers.

  D) The person who can identify existing and predictable hazards in the surroundings or working conditions which are unsanitary, hazardous, or dangerous to employees, and who has authorization to take prompt corrective measures to eliminate them.

13). The **PRIMARY** purpose of a job safety analysis (JSA) is to:

  A) Replace job instructions or workplace procedures.

  B) Document employee's accountability for their behavior.

  C) Review job methods, evaluate hazards, and identify controls.

  D) Demonstrate actively caring by management.

14). Which of the following will produce the **MOST** effective safety and health interface with contractors?

  A) The sub-contractor should develop their own procedures and follow them to the letter.

  B) The sub-contractor should use the general contractor's procedures to provide site standardization.

  C) The sub-contractor should follow all OSHA rules and, thus, will not need procedures.

  D) The sub-contractor should develop their own procedures with assistance from general contractor.

15). You are a newly hired supervisor on a job site. The person in the workplace with the most knowledge about how to accomplish a task is generally:

A) The worker.
B) The CEO.
C) General Manager.
D) The supervisor.

16). Who is required to provide placards when offering the shipment of a hazardous material?

A) The driver.
B) The carrier.
C) The shipper.
D) The manufacturer.

17). Fire is a hazard for many work activities and environments. A fire requires a chain reaction which includes:

A) Ignition, air and vapor.
B) Oxygen, fuel and heat.
C) Combustion, fuel and oxygen.
D) Air, vapor and fuel.

18). The three distinct parts of a "means of egress" are?

A) Exit access, exit, and exit discharge.
B) Door, passageway, and ramps.
C) Door opening device, door, and exit light.
D) Horizontal exits, stairs, and ramps.

19). A Commercial Motor Vehicle, transporting hazardous materials, is required to display placards in which of the following locations?

A) Front, rear and both sides of vehicle.
B) Front, rear and both sides of HAZMAT container.
C) Front, rear, top and both sides of vehicle.
D) Front, rear, top and both sides of HAZMAT container.

20). All the following are required on a confined space permit **EXCEPT**:

   A) The permit space to be entered.
   B) The purpose of the entry.
   C) The name of the CEO or President.
   D) The date and the authorized duration of the entry permit.

21). The **FIRST** step in emergency management planning is to:

   A) Identify and evaluate potential disasters.
   B) Assess potential harm that may be caused.
   C) Evaluate how many company assets are required.
   D) Decide on chain of command.

22). The **MOST** important reason for investigating mishaps is:

   A) To assess responsibility.
   B) To prevent future occurrences.
   C) For liability protection.
   D) For workers' compensation

23). The **PRIMARY** consideration when preparing for a potential disaster is?

   A) Selecting the emergency committee.
   B) Identifying a person to be the on-scene commander.
   C) Doing advanced emergency planning.
   D) Having a list of necessary state and federal directives.

24). The **PRIMARY** consideration in storing chemicals is?

   A) Ventilation.
   B) Fire Suppression.
   C) Control of static.
   D) Segregation.

25). A container for gasoline should be:

   A) Glass with a funnel.
   B) Plastic with a spill preventative spout.
   C) Metal with UL specified non-spill cap.
   D) Metal with a plastic spout.

Self-Assessment Quiz 2 Answers

1)   Answer C.

Accident costs have, for many years, been divided into direct and indirect costs. Direct costs are those costs directly and often immediately associated with the accident such as: transportation of injured, medical services, days lost from work etc. Indirect costs would include: lost production, replacement of injured worker, costs of training a replacement etc. **The indirect costs associated with accidents rarely consider the effects of a mishap on family members.**

2)   Answer A.

The supervisor is the prime investigator in most industrial accidents. They are closest to the action, and are most familiar with the environment, resultant interactions and stresses that occur. Supervisors are positioned in exactly the right position to provide valuable insight into the process which caused the accident, and to recommend corrective action to remedy the problem. Strangely enough, these are also the very same reasons the supervisor is not the correct person to do an in-depth investigation that will produce long lasting corrective actions. The supervisor is personally involved in the operation. He or she probably has friends among the workers. The credibility of the supervisor's position is on the line during any accident investigation. Can the supervisor honestly conduct an investigation that will, in the final analysis, point out deficiencies in management or supervision? Can they take off the company hat and become an impartial critic of the system, or of themselves? Often the answer to these questions is a resounding **no**! However, in spite of these obvious conflicts, the job of routine accident investigation still falls on the supervisors more often than not in the industrial environment.

3)   Answer A.

Senior management should investigate:

- Fatal accidents

- Accidents with large losses or potential for large losses

- Mishaps that result or could result in adverse public reaction

Lower levels of supervision and the safety director/engineer should also be involved in these investigations. The safety engineer should act as the company resident expert in mishap investigation procedures and techniques, offering advice and possibly training to other members of the investigation team. Most progressive companies also provide a standardized accident investigation "system" to be used on all important or large mishap investigations. The systems are varied and take many forms. They may be as simple as a checklist of items to be examined with a cause and effect report format, or an extensive system that details the entire investigative effort from membership to analysis to formal reporting with corporate presentations.

4)   Answer A.

There is no doubt that an investigator's first task is to arrive at the scene safely. All responders are in a hurry to get to the scene of the accident, but cannot render assistance or perform an adequate investigation if they do not arrive safely. The job of a health and safety professional cannot start until the scene is secured, meaning that the injured are taken care of and the scene itself is made safe. If responders arrive prior to scene security, they run the risk of becoming part of the emergency services effort, making them part of the response, rather than part of the investigative team. There are exceptions, such as in the case of the safety engineer who is part of a rescue or re-entry team, but in most cases, safe arrival to the scene is paramount.

5)   Answer B.

Dealing with hostile, belligerent or dishonest witnesses or participants, is a way of life for accident investigators. There are many theories about obtaining frank, candid and honest statements from these people. However, it is generally accepted that the most effective way is to explain that your investigation is for accident prevention purposes only and cannot be used for any type of disciplinary action. This tends to set the person at ease and will usually result in more open and honest responses about the mishap. However, investigators must be sure that they are telling the truth about purposes of the report. Often statements made in safety investigations wind up in personnel files or personnel action documents. Thus, assurance that investigative reports are only used for accident prevention purposes is essential. Do not provide false guarantees regarding. Develop a policy concerning safety investigation prior to the need!

6) Answer B.

This is a difficult question because the preferred place to conduct interviews changes with conditions. The investigator needs to make sure the witness feels at ease during the interview, which may mean conducting the interview at a location where the witness feels comfortable. However, the selected interview site must also provide privacy. Often the ideal place to interview witnesses is at the accident scene itself. This allows the witness a visual reference, fosters understanding and aids memory. Witnesses should always be interviewed individually to ensure unbiased reporting.

7) Answer B.

Often if evidence is to be used in a court of law, the chain of custody must be documented. The chain of custody is simply a documented explanation of where the evidence was obtained and where it has been since that time. The evidence must have been secured from tampering or alteration of any kind. The court must be assured through the chain of custody that the evidence has not been tampered with, or, if so, changes can be explained.

8) Answer C.

Prompt investigation of the accident scene, including interviewing witnesses, is of utmost importance; however, protection of the injured and prevention of a second accident must always take priority.

9) Answer D.

Accidents are usually multi-causal in nature and cannot be attributed entirely too any single factor.

10) Answer A.

De-energize: To free from any electric connection and/or electric charge.

Guarding: Placement of live parts of electrical equipment where they cannot accidentally be contacted, such as in a vault, behind a shield, or on a raised platform, to which only qualified persons have access.

Grounding: To prevent the buildup of hazardous voltages in a circuit by creating a low-resistance path to earth or some other ground plane.

11)   Answer D.

Collars, couplings, cams, clutches, flywheels, shaft ends, spindles, meshing gears, and horizontal or vertical shafting are some examples of common rotating mechanisms which may be hazardous. The basic types of hazardous mechanical motions and actions are:

Motions	Actions
Rotating	Cutting
In-Running Nip Points	Punching
Reciprocating	Shearing
Transversing	Bending

(2007). OSHA Machine Guarding eTool. *OSHA Machine Guarding eTool*. Retrieved OSHA-Machine Guarding eTool

12)   Answer D.

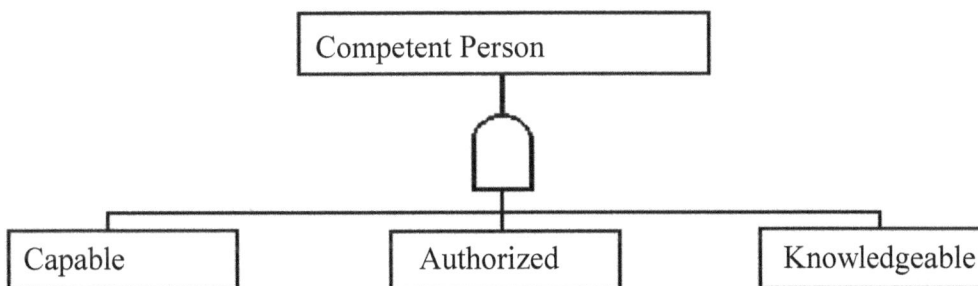

OSHA defines a competent person as "one who is capable of identifying existing and predictable hazards in the surroundings or working conditions which are unsanitary, hazardous, or dangerous to employees, and who has authorization to take prompt corrective measures to eliminate them". Additionally, the competent person should be a person who has extensive knowledge/experience in a particular activity or job function.

The result is a system fed by an "and" gate. The competent person must be capable "and" authorized "and" knowledgeable. Failure of any one of these elements results in failure of the entire system.

The use of a competent person is used often in many different OSHA construction standards including; lead, rigging, welding, fall protection, training, cranes and derricks, personnel hoisting, excavations, lift-slabs, steel erection, underground construction, compressed air, demolition, ladders, asbestos, cadmium etc. However, the definition is the same in all instances.

13)   Answer C.

Job Safety Analysis is a systematic analysis of job elements. It results in an in-depth evaluation by workers and first line supervisors of the individual steps and hazards. JSAs also offer protective measures or solutions to identified hazards. The principle benefits of a Job Safety Analysis (JSA) are as follows:

- Allowing the supervisor to perform training in safe, efficient operations

- Allowing the supervisor or other person developing the JSA to meet and work with employees

- Instructing new employees on specific jobs

- Instructing current employees on job specifics performed irregularly

- Acting as an accident investigation tool, should a mishap occur

- Studying jobs to determine if improvement is possible

14)   Answer D.

The current opinion is that the sub-contractors should develop their own procedures, with help from the general contractor. This method will assure maximum standardization and flexibility, while assuring effective accident prevention programs. This interface is not only effective, but helps each party to understand each other's concerns and allows both sides to develop better programs. Blind adherence to general contractors' programs usually does not work and causes further problems. For example, the requirement of a general contractor to use a particular type of fall protection or hardhat or eye protection may cause hardship for the sub-contractor. On the other hand, the use of a standardized general class of fall protection, or head protection is going to be required by general contractors, so some collaboration will be required. That is, the sub-contractor probably cannot follow procedures to the letter, so sub-contractors and general contractors should establish basic rules that all people involved can live with.

15)   Answer A.

The worker that performs the task is usually the most knowledgeable person about what is involved in accomplishing the task, issues that occur in doing a task and things that might affect performing the task. The worker that does the task should be the most knowledgeable, a new worker or new task would be an exception. Each worker should be adequately trained to perform a task safely as determined by the employer. This is the definition of competency.

16)   Answer C.

According to DOT regulations in 49 CFR Part 397, the shipper must:

- Transport the products by truck, railroad, ship or airplane
- Determine the product's proper shipping name, hazard class, identification number, correct packaging, placard, tables and markings
- Package materials, label and mark packages, prepare shipping paper and supply placards
- Certify on shipping paper that shipper properly complied with shipment rules.

17)   Answer B.

The traditional fire triangle theory states that there must be oxygen, fuel and heat for a fire to occur. Fuel cannot burn without an oxidizing agent and heat is required for ignition. The modern fire tetrahedron model recognizes the need for a chemical reaction to occur.

18)   Answer A.

NFPA 101, Life Safety Code, states, "A means of egress is a continuous and unobstructed way of exit travel from any point in a building or structure to a public way and consists of three separate and distinct parts: (a) the exit access, (b) the exit, and (c) the exit discharge. A means of egress comprises the vertical and horizontal travel and shall include intervening room spaces, doorways, hallways, corridors, passageways, balconies, ramps, stairs, enclosures, lobbies, escalators, horizontal exits, courts, and yards. It does **not** include elevators.

19)   Answer A.

According to 49 CFR 172.504, placards should be attached as workers load and before they drive the vehicle. The placards must appear on both sides and ends of the vehicle. Each placard must be

- Easily seen from direction it faces

- Placed so words or numbers are level and read from left to right

- At least three inches from other markings.

20)   Answer C.

1910.146(f) Entry permit: The entry permit that documents compliance with this section and authorizes entry to a permit space shall identify:

- Permit space to be entered;

- Purpose of the entry; Date and the authorized duration of the entry permit;

- Authorized entrants within the permit space, by name or by such other means (for example, through the use of rosters or tracking systems) as will enable the attendant to determine quickly and accurately, for the duration of the permit, which authorized entrants are inside the permit space.

NOTE: This requirement may be met by inserting a reference on the entry permit as to the means used, such as a roster or tracking system, to keep track of the authorized entrants within the permit space.

- Personnel, by name, currently serving as attendants

- Individual, by name, currently serving as entry supervisor, with a space for signature or initials of entry supervisor who originally authorized entry

- Hazards of permit space to be entered

- Measures used to isolate permit space and to eliminate or control permit space hazards before entry

NOTE: Those measures can include the lockout or tagging of equipment and procedures for purging, inerting, ventilating, and flushing permit spaces.

- Acceptable entry conditions

- Results of initial and periodic tests performed under paragraph (d)(5) of this section, accompanied by names or initials of testers and by an indication of when tests were performed

21) Answer A.

Although all answers need to be addressed during the planning process, according to the NSC, "before an organization initiates an emergency plan, it should identify and evaluate the potential disasters that might occur". During the follow of this process, you may have to develop mutual aid agreement with other companies or agencies in order to mitigate the emergencies or disasters.

22) Answer B:

Investigations should be performed to identify root causes and contributory causes in an effort to prevent reoccurrence of the accident.

23) Answer C:

According to the NSC, "advanced emergency management planning is the best way to minimize potential loss from natural or human caused disasters or accidents."

24) Answer D:

The first principle of good storage practice for chemicals is segregation, including separation from other materials in storage, from processing and handling operations and from incompatible materials.

1926.152(b) "Indoor storage of flammable and combustible liquids.": No more than 25 gallons of flammable or combustible liquids shall be stored in a room outside of an approved storage cabinet.

Quantities of flammable and combustible liquid in excess of 25 gallons shall be stored in an acceptable or approved cabinet meeting the following requirements:

Acceptable wooden storage cabinets shall be constructed in the following manner, or equivalent: The bottom, sides, and top shall be constructed of an exterior grade of plywood at least 1 inch in thickness, which shall not break down or delaminate under standard fire test conditions. All joints shall be rabbeted and shall be fastened in two directions with flathead wood screws. When more than one door is used, there shall be a rabbeted overlap of not less than 1 inch. Steel hinges shall be mounted in such a manner as to not lose their holding capacity due to loosening or burning out of screws when subjected to fire. Such cabinets shall be painted inside and out with fire retardant paint.

Approved metal storage cabinets will be acceptable. Cabinets shall be labeled in conspicuous lettering, "Flammable-Keep Fire Away." Not more than 60 gallons of flammable or 120 gallons of combustible liquids shall be stored in any one storage cabinet. Not more than three such cabinets may be in a single storage area. Quantities more than this shall be stored in an inside storage room.

25)   Answer C.

A UL approved container of 5 gallons or less with a spring-closed lid, spout cover, and flame arresting screen is commonly referred to as a safety can.

Self-Assessment Quiz 3 Questions

1). Personal protective equipment is crucial during welding and cutting operations. Which of the following statements is **MOST** correct concerning the proper shade of filter lens to use during welding & cutting operations?

    A) Generally, it is best to pick a #2 lens (dark) and work up, allows compensation for individual differences.

    B) The proper shade of filter lens should be matched to the type of welding and cutting operation.

    C) Heavy gas cutting would require a number 14 to 16 shade lens.

    D) It is usually best to start with a lens that gives a clear view of the weld zone and then move up.

2). The three types of scheduled safety inspections are:

    A) Monthly, quarterly, annually.

    B) Periodic, intermittent, general.

    C) Cross-functional, department specific, area specific.

    D) Third party, site specific, corporate.

3). A bench grinder should have the tool rest adjusted to within _____ inch of the wheel, and the tongue guard should be adjusted to within _____ inch of the wheel.

    A) 1/2 inch - 1/2 inch.

    B) 1/4 inch - 1/8 inch.

    C) 1/8 inch - 1/4 inch.

    D) 1/16 inch - 1/4 inch.

4). Proper procedure for inspection of chains during a semi-annual inspection is to:

    A) Check links with a caliper and compare at least 10 links.

    B) Check for cracks in end links.

    C) Compare twist on end sections.

    D) Perform a detailed link-by-link inspection of entire chain.

5). Level "B" Personal Protective Equipment (PPE) is defined as?

    A) Fully-encapsulated chemical-resistant suit with Self Contained Breathing Apparatus (SCBA) or Supplied Air (SA) with escape provisions.

    B) Chemical-resistant suit with Self Contained Breathing Apparatus (SCBA) or Supplied Air (SA) with escape provisions .

    C) Chemical-resistant suit with Air Purifying Respirator (APR).

    D) No chemical protection and no respiratory protection.

6). Which is the **BEST** example of a personal fall arrest system?

    A) Full body harness and lifeline attached to secure anchorage that limits the fall distance.

    B) An observer to warn workers when they approach the edge.

    C) Worker training on how to avoid a fall.

    D) Warning signs and demarcation of the access control zone.

7). During a heatstroke, which symptom(s) would a worker **UNLIKELY** experience?

    A) Severe headache.

    B) Profuse sweating and cool moist skin.

    C) Loss of consciousness.

    D) Rapid temperature rises and hot dry skin.

8). Employers should perform safety inspections_____?

    A) Once per day.

    B) Once per week.

    C) Frequently and regularly.

    D) As often as needed.

9). A STSC observes the back of a rough terrain fork truck lift off the ground as a heavy load is being lifted on a job site. Which of the following is the **FIRST** course of action?

    A) Direct the crew to add extra counter weight to stabilize the operation.

    B) Stop the crew and advise to discontinue with the lift.

    C) Instruct the crew to add air to load side tires.

    D) Direct the operator to tip mast back once load is lifted.

10). **MINIMALLY**, all guardrail systems shall be capable of withstanding, without failure, a force of at least _____ pounds applied within 2 inches (5.1 cm) of the top edge, in any outward or downward direction, at any point along the top edge.

    A) 150 pounds.
    B) 200 pounds.
    C) 210 pounds.
    D) 240 pounds.

11). The **PRIMARY** reason for accident investigation of occupational safety and health issues is?
    A) To determine facts surrounding the event.
    B) To establish who or what was at fault.
    C) To determine obvious cause factors.
    D) To establish a baseline for further analysis.

12). A worker arrives on site with own personal protective equipment (PPE). Who is responsible to ensure the PPE is appropriate for the job?

    A) Employer.
    B) Employee.
    C) PPE manufacturer.
    D) Union representative.

13). Which of the following are the two categories used to identify respiratory protection?
    A) Particulate and Supplied Air.
    B) Self-cleaning and Non-self-cleaning.
    C) Air-purifying and Air-supplied.
    D) Gas Masks and Air Hoods.

14). A modern management approach to the success of a long-term safety management system is known as?

    A) Micro management.
    B) Creating silos.
    C) Team-based.
    D) Employee enforcement.

15). The horizontal distance from base to vertical plane of support in straight ladder placement should be approximately _____ the ladder length between supports.

     A) 1/3
     B) 1/4
     C) 1/2
     D) 1/8

16). A worker arrives at work with his own sunglasses stating they are "safe enough." His supervisor should look for:

     A) Markings for ANSI Z87 on frame.
     B) Proper light refraction in lenses by holding to light.
     C) Nothing. Allow worker to wear sunglasses.
     D) Nothing. Have worker check with Site Manager.

17). A skin cancer caused by sunlight exposure is called?

     A) Mesothelioma.
     B) Sarcomas.
     C) Leukemia.
     D) Melanoma.

18). The **BEST** descriptor of the barrier cream function is:

     A) Replace lanolin in skin.
     B) Keep hands clean.
     C) Inhibit contact of solvent with skin surface.
     D) Provide a cure for chapped, dry hands and feet.

19). Which controls are listed in order of decreasing effectiveness, **MOST to LEAST** effective, to prevent industrial dermatitis?

     A) Gloves, signage, industrial hygiene, elimination.
     B) Chemical substitution, procedures, gloves, barrier cream.
     C) Face shields, procedures, signage, ventilation.
     D) Splash shields, chemical substitution, barrier cream, gloves.

20). Which type of radiation from welding operations is the **MOST** damaging to the eyes?

    A) Light.
    B) Ultraviolet.
    C) Infrared.
    D) Visible light.

21). What is the effect that high humidity has on the service life of a cartridge respirator?

    A) Cartridge respirators are not for use in high humidity environments.
    B) To decrease the service life.
    C) To have no impact on the service life.
    D) To increase the service life.

22). Which of the following is the **LEAST important** role of front line supervision in a successful safety program?

    A) Provide daily training.
    B) Know the workplace and work.
    C) Protect their employees from potential hazards.
    D) Write safety procedures.

23). Which of the following factors **does NOT** affect the load capacity of a mobile crane?

    A) Boom length.
    B) Boom angle.
    C) Extension of outriggers.
    D) Installation of anti-two-blocking device.

24). Written safety programs should be written in:

    A) English.
    B) Language of management.
    C) Language of workers.
    D) Language of both management and workers.

25). Workers must be trained on all hazardous chemicals:

    A) In their work area.
    B) At home.
    C) On site.
    D) Used by each contractor crew.

Self-Assessment Quiz 3 Answers

1) Answer B.

Proper eye protection is among the most important safety precautions welders and metal cutters can take. The proper shade protection is very important to guard against the damage caused by UV and IR radiation created during these operations. The table shown here was taken directly from the OSHA standards. Additional information is contained in ANSI/ASC Z49.1-88.

OSHA 1926.102 Table E-2 Filter Lens Shade Numbers For Protection Against Radiant Energy

Welding Operation	Shade Number
Shielded metal-arc welding 1/16, 3/32, 1/8, 5/32 inch diameter electrodes	10
Gas-shielded arc welding (nonferrous) 1/16, 3/32, 1/8, 5/32 inch diameter electrodes	11
Gas-shielded arc welding (ferrous) 1/16, 3/32, 1/8, 5/32 inch diameter electrodes	12
Shielded metal-arc welding 3/16, 7/32, 1/4 inch diameter electrodes	12
5/16, 3/8 inch diameter electrodes	14
Atomic hydrogen welding	10-14
Carbon-arc welding	14
Soldering	2
Torch brazing	3 or 4
Light cutting, up to 1 inch	3 or 4
Medium cutting, 1 inch to 6 inches	4 or 5
Heavy cutting, over 6 inches	5 or 6
Gas welding (light), up to 1/8 inch	4 or 5
Gas welding (medium), 1/8 inch to 1/2 inch	5 or 6
Gas welding (heavy), over 1/2 inch	6 or 8

2)   Answer C.

According to the National Safety Council's Supervisors' Safety Manual, there are three types of scheduled inspections:

- Periodic inspections are inspections of specific items conducted daily, weekly, monthly, quarterly, annually or at any given intervals.
- Intermittent (special) inspections or assessments are performance at irregular intervals or for cause.
- General inspections are designed to include all areas that do not receive periodic inspections.

3)   Answer C.

According to the National Safety Council's "Accident Prevention Manual for Industrial Operations", tool rests should be adjusted to not more than 1/8 inch from the grinding wheel tongue guards should be adjusted to 1/4 inch.

4)   Answer D.

Chain inspections should be done visually in an attempt to detect any elongation or other defect. This is best accomplished by a link-by-link inspection. Overall measurements or caliper readings of a section are often misleading because not all links will be affected or damaged.

5)   Answer B.

Modified Chart of EPA/OSHA Levels of Protection			
Levels	Skin	Respiratory	When
A	Fully-encapsulating, chemical-resistant suit, inner gloves, chemical-resistant safety boots.	Pressure-demand, full-facepiece SCBA or pressure-demand supplied-air respirator with escape SCBA.	Highest level of protection indicated by high concentration of atmospheric vapors, gases or particulates or splash hazard exists.

B	Chemical-resistant clothing (overalls and long-sleeved jacket; hooded, one or two piece chemical splash suit; disposable chemical-resistant one-piece suit), inner and outer gloves, chemical resistant safety boots and hard hat.	Pressure-demand, full-facepiece SCBA or pressure-demand supplied-air respirator with escape SCBA.	High level of respiratory protection required, but less skin protection. IDLH, less than 19.5% oxygen.
C	Chemical-resistant clothing (overalls and long-sleeved jacket; hooded, one or two piece chemical splash suit; disposable chemical-resistant one-piece suit), inner and outer gloves, chemical resistant safety boots and hard hat.	Full-facepiece, air-purifying, canister-equipped respirator.	The contaminants, splashes, or direct contact will not affect exposed flesh. Canister will remove contaminant.
D	Overalls, Safety Boots, safety glasses or chemical splash goggles, hardhat.	No respiratory protection and minimal skin protection.	The atmosphere contains no known hazard. Splashes, immersion or inhalation improbable

6)   Answer A.

Employers must set up the work place to prevent employees from falling off of overhead platforms, elevated work stations or into holes in the floor and walls. OSHA requires that fall protection be provided at elevations of four feet in general industry workplaces, five feet in shipyards, six feet in the construction industry and eight feet in longshoring operations. In addition, OSHA requires that fall protection be provided when working over dangerous equipment and machinery, regardless of the fall distance.

To prevent employees from being injured from falls, employers must:

- Guard every floor hole into which a worker can accidentally walk (using a railing and toe-board or a floor hole cover).
- Provide a guard rail and toe-board around every elevated open sided platform, floor or runway, stair railings and hand rails.
- Regardless of height, if a worker can fall into or onto dangerous machines or equipment (such as a vat of acid or a conveyor belt) employers must provide guardrails and toe-boards to prevent workers from falling and getting injured.
- Fall protection that may be required on certain jobs include safety harness and line, 5000 lbs per person anchor points, safety nets, calculated fall distance and rescue plans.

7)   Answer B.

During heatstroke (sunstroke), the body temperature rises and reaches a point where the heat-regulating mechanism breaks down completely. The body temperature then rises rapidly. The symptoms include hot dry skin, severe headache, visual disturbances, rapid temperature rise, and loss of consciousness.

8)   Answer C.

Well managed inspection programs will exist at several levels where hazard prevention and control are managed best. They have many purposes, one of the most important being that they display and communicate management's determination that hazardous conditions and practices are to be identified and corrected while positive safety performance is recognized. Inspections provide meaningful opportunities for participation and should be performed frequently and regularly.

9)   Answer B.

A fork truck should never be operated with an overload. This condition removes weight from the steering wheels, which affects control of the machine. Never add counterweight because it can seriously overload the forks, tires, axles, chains etc.

10)   Answer B.

1926.502(b)

"Guardrail systems." Guardrail systems and their use shall comply with the following provisions:

- Top edge height of top rails, or equivalent guardrail system members, shall be 42 inches (1.1 m) plus or minus 3 inches (8 cm) above the walking/working level. When conditions warrant, the height of the top edge may exceed the 45-inch height, provided the guardrail system meets all other criteria of this paragraph.

- **Note**: When employees are using stilts, the top edge height of the top rail, or equivalent member, shall be increased an amount equal to the height of the stilts.

- Midrails, screens, mesh, intermediate vertical members, or equivalent intermediate structural members shall be installed between the top edge of the guardrail system and the walking/working surface when there is no wall or parapet wall at least 21 inches (53 cm) high.

- Midrails, when used, shall be installed at a height midway between the top edge of the guardrail system and the walking/working level.

- Screens and mesh, when used, shall extend from the top rail to the walking/working level and along the entire opening between top rail supports.

Intermediate members (such as balusters), when used between posts, shall be not more than 19 inches (48 cm) apart.

Other structural members (such as additional midrails and architectural panels) shall be installed such that there are no openings in the guardrail system that are more than 19 inches (0.5 m) wide.

Guardrail systems shall be capable of withstanding, without failure, a force of at least 200 pounds (890 N) applied within 2 inches (5.1 cm) of the top edge, in any outward or downward direction, at any point along the top edge.

11)   Answer A.

According to the National Safety Council, accident investigation should be conducted to provide the facts. If fault-finding is attempted, the investigation may cause more harm than good. Mishap investigation is conducted to determine both obvious and hidden cause factors. It does tend to serve as the baseline for further analysis, but selection "A" is the *primary* reason for investigation.

12)   Answer A.

The employer is responsible for conducting a PPE assessment and ensuring that the proper PPE is worn.

13)   Answer C.

All respirators can be placed in two categories: air purifying or air supplying

14)   Answer C.

A Team-based approach to safety management is a modern management model used to continuously improve a safety management system.

15)   Answer B.

When setting up a straight ladder, the base should be one-fourth the ladder length from the vertical plane of the top support.

16)   Answer A.

ANSI approves specifications for safety glasses. The markings for ANSI Z87 on frames are the indicator that they meet ANSI standards for impact lenses.

17)   Answer D.

Sunlight is the most common occupational cause of melanoma skin cancer.

18)   Answer C.

Protective creams, sometimes called "Barrier" creams, serve to inhibit contact with solvents in the work place. The use of protective creams is very controversial, however, most current Safety and Health literature indicates, when used properly, these creams are useful. The cream must be used correctly to be effective, which means it must be applied on clean skin at the beginning of the work shift, removed at lunch, reapplied after lunch, again in the afternoon, and removed at work shift end.

19)   Answer B.

It is generally accepted within the safety and health industry that substitution is the most effective control method for industrial dermatosis prevention. Substitution is followed by gloves and barrier cream. Good hygiene practice is, of course, required in all industrial settings.

20)   Answer C.

Both Ultraviolet (UV) and Infrared radiation (IR) will cause damage to the eyes. However, IR is very penetrating and passes through the cornea to the retina of the eye causing permanent damage. Ultraviolet radiation will cause eye burn (Arc Eye) that is painful and disabling but, signs and symptoms usually disappear in 12 to 36 hours and, as stated earlier, are confined to the cornea.

21)   Answer B.

Relative Humidity is a measure of the amount of water vapor the air will hold at a specified temperature and is   expressed in percentage values. Since warmer air will hold more water than colder air, the same relative humidity at a higher temperature represents a significantly greater amount of moisture. High relative humidity is a significant negative factor in the capacity of organic vapor cartridges since the large quantity of water vapor will compete with the organic vapors for active sites on the adsorbent. Most of the laboratory work determining adsorbent capacity has been performed at a low relative humidity of 50% at approximately 70°F.

 (OSHA, 1998) Retrieved OSHA-Respiratory Protection eTool

22)   Answer D.

Writing safety procedures can be important, however, is the least important role of those listed in the question.

23)   Answer D.

Installation of anti-two-blocking device does not affect the load capacity of a mobile crane.

24)   Answer D.

Best practice with a multicultural and multilingual workforce is to present information in the language of both management and workers. This may include the use of key safety words, phrases, and pictograms.

25)   Answer A.

OSHA's HAZCOM standard 1910.1200 states Employee training should include at least: Methods and observations that may be used to detect the presence or release of a hazardous chemical in the work area (such as monitoring conducted by the employer, continuous monitoring devices, appearance or odor of hazardous chemicals when being released, etc.); The physical and health hazards of the chemicals in the work area; The measures employees can take to protect themselves from these hazards, including specific procedures the employer has implemented to protect employees from exposure to hazardous chemicals, such as appropriate work practices, emergency procedures, and personal protective equipment to be used; and, The details of the hazard communication program to be developed by the employer, including an explanation of the labeling system and the material safety data sheet, and how employees can obtain and use the appropriate hazard information.

Self-Assessment Quiz 4 Questions

1). An engineer replaces steel clips with hot dip galvanized clips to weld. The welder asks the supervisor about the fumes from the galvanized clips. The supervisor should:

    A) Provide a respirator.
    B) Take breaks to not get overexposed.
    C) Drink milk and antacids to offset effects of galvanized fumes.
    D) Consult SDS for hot dip galvanized clips for protective measures.

2). A worker complains of feeling ill after an unknown layer of coating was found during a grinding operation. The Supervisor should:

    A) Have them keep working to see if the symptoms subside.
    B) Take an extra break during the task.
    C) Stop work until the coating can be identified.
    D) Replace the worker.

3). Another contracting crew is spraying hazardous materials in your crew's work area. Your company has a respirator program. Supervisor should:

    A) Continue working assuming the contractor will inform you if protective actions are needed.
    B) Determine the hazards of the materials being sprayed and take appropriate protective actions for the crew.
    C) Write report to site management.
    D) Give crew particulate respirators.

4). Accident costs such as loss in earning power, loss of time by supervision, damage to tools and equipment, and cost of training a new worker are also called?

    A) Direct costs.
    B) Insured costs.
    C) Indirect costs.
    D) Miscellaneous costs.

5). An employer must provide employees with information and training on hazardous chemicals in their work area **EXCEPT**:

    A) At the time, they are hired and assigned.
    B) Whenever a new physical or health hazard is introduced to their work area.
    C) On the day, they are transferred to a new job.
    D) When the chemicals are used below the exposure limit.

6). If a serious violation exists, and the CSHO finds that the supervisor had full knowledge of the hazard, does this constitute a serious violation?

    A) No, the supervisor is considered an employee, not the employer.
    B) Yes, the supervisor represents the employer and a supervisor's knowledge of the hazard amounts to employer knowledge.
    C) No, the supervisor could have chosen not to have told the owner.
    D) Yes, the owner should have known if he/she would have been doing his/her job.

7). During a periodic inspection of chains, the condition that **LEAST** affects metallurgic failure is:

    A) Bent links.
    B) Painted links.
    C) Corrosion pits in the links.
    D) Stretching caused by overloading.

8). It is **MOST** important to provide new employee training and orientation because:

    A) New employees are easier to train than employees who have been on the job longer.
    B) New employees are less likely to have accidents at work.
    C) New employees are inexperienced and not familiar with the hazards, procedures, facilities and safety rules.
    D) New employees tend to break rules to test the system.

9). Safety and health meetings are conducted **PRIMARILY** to?

   A) Discuss the work of the day.
   B) Motivate employees to take an interest and responsibility for safety and health.
   C) Train employees in risk reduction techniques.
   D) Allow employees to air their complaints.

10). The **BEST** method to control or eliminate a hazard is to?

   A) Use personal protective equipment (PPE).
   B) Utilize administrative controls.
   C) Utilize engineering controls.
   D) Display hazard warning signage.

11). The **BEST** ladder practice is to:

   A) Face the ladder when ascending or descending.
   B) Hold on with one hand when climbing while carrying material.
   C) Climb a ladder with muddy or greasy shoes.
   D) Slide down a ladder.

12). Enclosures for noise control are designed to:

   A) Isolate individual from noise source.
   B) Reduce noise level at source.
   C) Reduce worker exposure to noise.
   D) Increase distance between source and receiver.

13). The **BEST** approach for reducing incidents involving human error is to?

   A) Carefully screen job applicants.
   B) Furnish workers with PPE.
   C) Improve system design.
   D) Improve workplace conditions.

14). Incident investigations are primarily conducted to determine the causal factors. The person **MOST** responsible for implementing corrective actions is the:

    A) Frontline Supervisor.
    B) Safety Manager.
    C) Facilities Manager.
    D) Quality Manager.

15). The **LEAST** appropriate purpose for accident (mishap) investigation is for:

    A) Preventing reoccurrence of similar events.
    B) Establishing causal factors.
    C) Providing vehicle for discipline.
    D) Providing data for trend analysis.

16). Who is responsible to ensure an employee's personal PPE is used properly?

    A) Employee.
    B) PPE manufacturer.
    C) Union representative.
    D) Supervisor.

17). A respirator with a filter, cartridge, or canister element that removes specific air contaminants is termed:

    A) An air-purifying respirator.
    B) A positive filter respirator.
    C) A negative pressure respirator.
    D) An air-supplying respirator.

18). Which of the following **BEST** describes an expectation of the STS Code of Ethics?

    A) Perform their supervisory roles in a manner to protect their employer.

    B) Perform their safety roles using their knowledge and skills to further the safety of employees, employers, the public and the environment.

    C) Avoid circumstances that might compromise their employer or their employees.

    D) Maintain confidentiality of all information that might impugn their employer or client.

19). The **MOST** important purpose for supervisor involvement with incident investigation is?

    A) Immediate supervisors are usually the most knowledgeable about the work.

    B) Immediate supervisors have limited responsibility in the safety of their workers and are, therefore, more objective investigators.

    C) Immediate supervisors know the injured person's family best.

    D) Immediate supervisors are usually not involved with correcting the problem.

20). All lanyards and vertical lifelines have a minimum breaking strength of _____ pounds per worker.

    A) 1000

    B) 2000

    C) 5000

    D) 10,000

21). The **MAXIMUM** storage temperature for a gas cylinder is:

    A) 100° F

    B) 100° C

    C) 130° F

    D) 130° C

22). The **FIRST** item to complete before rigging a sling to a load is to:

A) Load test the sling at 150% of rated capacity.
B) The rated load capacity for the sling.
C) Inspect the sling after use.
D) Inspect sling weekly.

23). The action **MOST** likely to produce severe injuries or a high probability of accidents is:

A) Routine tasks.
B) Volunteer tasks.
C) Closely supervised actions.
D) Unusual and non-routine tasks.

24). A standard railing shall consist of top rail, intermediate rail, and posts, and shall have a vertical height of ___ inches nominal from upper surface of top rail to floor, platform, runway, or ramp level.

A) 36
B) 40
C) 42
D) 48

25). Job site safety training is a critical part of a safety program. Which of the following statements is most true?

A) While comprehensive, pre-assignment training covering company assigned topics is necessary, all workers perform best when allowed to self-study training materials.
B) While comprehensive, pre-assignment training covering regulatory required topics is necessary, on the job experience is the best "trainer." Until workers make their own mistakes, they won't really learn.
C) Comprehensive, pre-assignment training covering all needed topics and information is the best method of ensuring employees are trained and qualified to perform their tasks safely.
D) While comprehensive, pre-assignment training covering regulatory required topics is necessary, short, single topic tailgate meetings are very effective.

Self-Assessment Quiz 4 Answers

1)   Answer D.

The best answer is to consult with the Safety Data Sheet (SDS) for worker protection information. According to SDS, during welding operations with galvanized clips, the supervisor should provide adequate ventilation and appropriate particulate respirator to protect against metal fumes. Zinc is used in large quantities in the manufacture of brass, galvanized metals, and various other alloys. Inhalation of zinc oxide fumes can occur when welding or cutting on zinc-coated metals. Exposure to these fumes is known to cause metal fume fever. Symptoms of metal fume fever are very similar to those of common influenza. They include fever (rarely exceeding 102° F), chills, nausea, dryness of the throat, cough, fatigue, and general weakness and aching of the head and body. The victim may sweat profusely for a few hours, after which the body temperature begins to return to normal. The symptoms of metal fume fever have rarely, if ever, lasted beyond 24 hours.

2)   Answer C.

Anytime there is an unknown suspected chemical exposure, accompanied by symptoms in workers, it is best to stop work and determine how to prevent exposure.

3)   Answer B.

The supervisor must determine hazards of materials being sprayed and take appropriate protective actions for the crew.

4)   Answer C.

Accident costs such as loss in earning power, loss of time by supervision, damage to tools and equipment, and cost of training a new worker are also called indirect costs.

5)   Answer D.

Employees are to be trained at the time they are assigned to work with a hazardous chemical. The intent of this provision (1910.1200(h)) is to have information prior to exposure to prevent the occurrence of adverse health effects. This purpose cannot be met if training is delayed until a later date. The training provisions of the HCS are not satisfied solely by giving employee the data sheets to read. An employer's training program is to be a forum for explaining to employees not only the hazards of the chemicals in their work area, but also how to use the information generated in the hazard communication program. This can be accomplished in many ways (audiovisuals, classroom instruction, interactive video), and should include an opportunity for employees to ask questions to ensure that they understand the information presented to them. Training need not be conducted on each specific chemical found in the workplace, but may be conducted by categories of hazard (e.g., carcinogens, sensitizers, acutely toxic agents) that are or may be encountered by an employee during the course of his duties. Furthermore, the training must be comprehensible. If the employees receive job instructions in a language other than English, then the training and information to be conveyed under the HCS will also need to be conducted in a foreign language.

6)   Answer B.

The OSHAct Section 17 explains that: "a serious violation shall be deemed to exist in a place of employment if there is a substantial probability that death or serious physical harm could result from a condition which exists, or from one or more practices, means, methods, operations, or processes which have been adopted or are in use, in such place of employment unless the employer did not, and could not with the exercise of reasonable diligence, know of the presence of the violation."

In determining if a hazard is serious or not, the question was "**Whether the employer knew**, or with the exercise of reasonable diligence, could have known of the presence of the hazardous condition. In this regard, the supervisor represents the employer and a supervisor's knowledge of the hazardous condition amounts to employer knowledge. In cases where the employer may contend that the supervisor's own conduct constitutes an isolated event of employee misconduct, the CSHO will attempt to determine the extent to which the supervisor was trained and supervised to prevent such conduct, and how the employer enforces the rule. If, after reasonable attempts to do so, it cannot be determined that the employer has actual knowledge of the hazardous condition, the knowledge requirement is met in the eyes of OSHA, if the CSHO is satisfied that the employer could have known through exercise of reasonable diligence. As a general rule, if the CSHO was able to discover a hazardous condition, and the condition was not transitory in nature, it can be presumed that the employer could have discovered the same condition through the exercise of reasonable diligence.

7)   Answer B.

According to the National Safety Council, a link-by-link inspection should be made to detect the following:

- Bent links
- Cracks in weld areas, in shoulders or in any other section of link
- Transverse nicks or gouges
- Corrosion pits
- Stretching caused by overloading

8)   Answer C.

New employees are more likely to have accidents at work and may be inexperienced on the job site and not familiar with the hazards, safety procedure, facilities and safety rules and regulations.

9)   Answer B.

To motivate employees to take an interest and responsibility for safety and Health is the best answer. The safety committee can have many different functions, but it primarily represents employee involvement.

10)   Answer C.

Engineering controls are the best method to eliminate hazards.

11)   Answer A.

Workers should always face the ladder and have three points of contact on the ladder.

12) Answer B.

Generally, an enclosure is placed around a noise source to prevent noise from getting outside. Enclosures are normally lined with sound-absorption material to decrease internal sound pressure buildup.

13) Answer C.

Improving system design is the best solution for minimizing and eliminating human error.

14) Answer A.

The cause factors discovered during accident investigations are normally corrected by the level of supervision that exercises control over the operation.

15) Answer C.

Accident investigation has as its primary purpose the prevention of similar occurrences and the discovery of hazards. The intent is not to place blame or administer discipline, but rather to determine how responsibilities may be defined or clarified and to reduce error producing situations. Accident investigation should improve the safety of operations, if accident investigation is used for punitive measures, the tool has the reverse effect.

16) Answer D.

Employee-owned equipment: Where employees provide their own protective equipment, the employer shall be responsible to assure its adequacy, including proper maintenance, and sanitation of such equipment. The supervisor is generally tasked with ensuring PPE is worn properly.

17) Answer A.

Air-Purifying Respirator: A respirator with an air-purifying filter, cartridge, or canister that removes specific air contaminants by passing ambient air through the air-purifying element.

18) Answer B.

"Perform their safety roles using their knowledge and skills to further the safety of employees, employers, the public and the environment" best describes an expectation of the STS Code of Ethics.

19) Answer A.

Immediate supervisors are (normally) the most knowledgeable of the work and have a major responsibility in safety of their employees. Therefore, they should be the ones who are most concerned about correcting problems, thus, preventing other incidents, i.e., near misses, injuries, etc.

20) Answer C.

Lanyards and vertical lifelines shall have a minimum breaking strength of 5,000 pounds (22.2 kN).

21) Answer C.

Cylinders are not designed for temperatures in excess of 130 degrees F or 54 degrees C.

22) Answer B.

Verify that the rated load capacity for the rope or sling is being exceeded.

23) Answer D.

Unusual and non-routine tasks are more likely to result in injuries than the other choices.

24)   Answer C.

A standard railing shall consist of top rail, intermediate rail, and posts, and shall have a vertical height of 42 inches nominal from upper surface of top rail to floor, platform, runway, or ramp level. The top rail shall be smooth-surfaced throughout the length of the railing. The intermediate rail shall be approximately halfway between the top rail and the floor, platform, runway, or ramp. The ends of the rails shall not overhang the terminal posts, except where such overhang does not constitute a projection hazard.

A standard toe board shall be 4 inches nominal in vertical height from its top edge to the level of the floor, platform, runway, or ramp. It shall be securely fastened in place and with not more than 1/4-inch clearance above floor level. It may be made of any substantial material, either solid or with openings, not over 1 inch in greatest dimension.

25)   Answer D.

Safety training is a crucial part of a comprehensive safety program. There are many topics that regulations require training to be accomplished prior to job assignment. Industry has recognized that ongoing training provided for short periods of time (less than an hour), covering single topics is a very effective method to training workers. The key to safety training is to provide workers with information to prevent accidents and injuries.

Self-Assessment Quiz 5 Questions

1). When training workers in erecting and dismantling scaffolding, which statement is **MOST** correct?

    A) Training must be done by a Certified Safety, Health and Environmental Trainer (CET).
    B) A scaffold competent person must conduct the training.
    C) Training is not required for scaffold assembly nor dismantling.
    D) Training is a good practice and is not required by regulations.

2). What is the **MOST** important consideration during the planning stage of a Health & Safety Training Program?

    A) Training Objectives.
    B) Training Methods.
    C) Instructor Qualifications.
    D) Training Program Content.

3). Immediate feedback on crew performance is **MOST** routinely provided by the:

    A) First line supervisor.
    B) General Superintendent.
    C) Project Manager/General Manager.
    D) Safety and Health Representative.

4). **MOST** eye injuries at work are a result of?

    A) Corrosive substances.
    B) Weld burns.
    C) Flying objects.
    D) Gases and vapors.

5). Which statement is **INCONSISTANT** with the STS Code of Ethics and Professional Conduct?

    A) STS certificate holders should use their knowledge and skill for enhancement of safety and health of employees, employers, and public, as well as environment and property.

    B) STS certificate holders should strive to increase their own competence and integrity and honor of the profession.

    C) STS certificate holders should represent their profession and certification in an honest forthright manner.

    D) STS certificate holders should endeavor to represent the common good of the public, without respect to the needs of employers or clients.

6). What is the cause of **MOST** accidents?

    A) A specific unsafe act.
    B) Many contributing causes.
    C) A condition in the field.
    D) Poor supervision.

7). The **LEAST** effective time to present a safety training session is after?
    A) An accident
    B) The company announces it is downsizing
    C) The monthly accident data shows an increase in incident rate
    D) A plant explosion

8). This training method is **PRIMARILY** used to find new, innovative approaches to issues.

    A) Meeting
    B) Brainstorming
    C) Case Study
    D) Role Playing

9). Of the following, the **LEAST** important benefit of safety and health training is:

    A) Improved performance
    B) Fewer accidents
    C) Reduced costs
    D) Attitude adjustment

10). A supervisor's company has hired a new worker who was qualified as a powered truck operator at her previous company. What is the training required to get this person qualified as a power truck operator in the company?

    A) Send to a formal school.
    B) Accept the other company's qualification.
    C) Have the employee attend your company's initial training program.
    D) Ensure the operator has knowledge and skills required to operate power trucks, including company's procedures.

11). On-the-Job training is **PRIMARILY** used because?

    A) It is cost effective.
    B) More than one person can be trained at a time.
    C) Requires minimum amount of time for total training.
    D) Allows workers to produce during training period.

12). Safety and health training should be targeted to real problems and only recommended as problem solutions where increased knowledge or skill is needed or required by directive. What is the **BEST** reason or objective for post-training observation?

    A) To weed out weak performers.
    B) To spot workers who have "attitude" problems.
    C) To evaluate if the training program objectives align with job performance.
    D) To determine if students liked the training.

13). The **BEST** indicator of training effectiveness is?

    A) Favorable student critiques.
    B) Correct student response to questions.
    C) Improved job performance.
    D) Testing meets expected norms.

14). A break in elevation of _____ requires that either steps, ramps, or ladders must be provided.

    A) 10 inches
    B) 18 inches
    C) 19 inches
    D) 12 inches

15). Which of the following would **NOT** require employers to provide employees training on hazardous chemicals in the workplace?

    A) Initial assignment
    B) Resupply of chemicals
    C) Change in job assignment with new chemicals
    D) New chemical hazard in work environment

16). When selecting extension cords for power tools the **MOST** appropriate considerations are:

    A) The power requirements, type of tool, and the wire gauge.
    B) The resistance, wire gauge, and length of run.
    C) The power requirements, wire gauge, and length of run
    D) The type of tool, the wire gauge, and wet areas.

17). In storage, gas cylinders must be separated from other combustible material by 20 feet or a barrier that is non-combustible, has a 30-minute fire rating and is at least _____ feet high?

    A) 3
    B) 5
    C) 7
    D) 10

18). Employees required to use PPE must be trained in all areas **EXCEPT**?

    A) How to purchase PPE.
    B) When PPE is necessary.
    C) Limitations of PPE.
    D) How to properly don, doff, adjust, and wear PPE.

19). One factor that does **NOT** contribute to the depletion of oxygen levels in confined spaces is?

   A) Chemical reaction.
   B) Welding.
   C) Bacterial action.
   D) Ventilation.

20). The individual in the **BEST** position to provide effective safety training of work groups is/are?

   A) Supervisors.
   B) Senior Management.
   C) New Hires.
   D) Training Professionals.

21). The main objective of Health and Safety communications with workers is **PRIMARILY** to?

   A) Teach workers to understand what is being said
   B) Provide a vehicle for suggestions
   C) Teach workers to write and read well
   D) Provide a safety message that will be understood and accepted by workers

22). Effective training is enhanced by using lesson plans which are designed to?

   A) Be provided as a course handout
   B) Provide the trainees with course objectives
   C) Provide the instructor with standardized guidance for training session
   D) For instructor and students to review prior to beginning of training session

23).   Communication is **BEST** defined as:

    A) Sharing information and/or ideas with others and being understood.
    B) Sharing information and/or ideas with others and gaining approval.
    C) Sharing opinions and/or ideas with others and being understood.
    D) Sharing opinions and/or ideas with others and gaining approval.

24).   The class of employees that has the **GREATEST** potential for accidents is:

    A) New employees.
    B) Experienced employees.
    C) Administrative employees.
    D) Disabled employees.

25).   Which communication technique is **MOST** effective in the workplace?

    A) Face to face group lecture.
    B) Face to face group two-way communications.
    C) Face to face individual two-way communications.
    D) Written individual two-way communications.

Self-Assessment Quiz 5 Answers

1)   Answer B.

OSHA requires a competent person to provide training on the nature of fall hazards, correct procedures for erection, maintenance and disassembly, proper use, placement and care in handling, etc.   Additionally, all erection and disassembly must be done under the supervision of a competent person.

2)   Answer A.

The establishment of Training Objectives is the key to good planning. No other single element has the ability to allow the training program to succeed.

3)   Answer A.

The positive feedback from a worker's immediate supervisor is the best form of recognition for good safety performance.

4)   Answer C.

Most commonly, an eye becomes scratched when a foreign body enters it and the individual then rubs the eye in an attempt to remove the irritation. Eyes also become scratched when they are poked by a foreign body. A scratched eye can become serious very quickly, with a fungal infection for example, so seeing a doctor if there is no improvement in a day or two is crucial. In addition, a scratched eye can be worse for individuals who wear contacts.

5)   Answer D.

Selection D is inconsistent with fundamental principles of the BCSP STS Code of Ethics and Professional Conduct.

STS certificate holders should endeavor to represent the common good of the public _**AND**_ the needs of employers and clients.

6)   Answer B.

Most accident investigations will reveal several direct and indirect causes.

7)   Answer B.

Events such as the company announces it is downsizing is not an ideal time to conduct safety training.

8)   Answer B.

Brainstorming is a technique of group interactions that encourages each participant to present ideas on a specific issue. The method is normally used to find new, innovative approaches to issues. There are four ground rules:

- Ideas presented are not criticized.
- Freewheeling creative thinking and building on ideas are positively reinforced.
- As many ideas as possible should be quickly presented.
- Combining several ideas or improving suggestions is encouraged.

9)   Answer D.

The benefits of safety and health training include all the following except:
- Improved performance
- Fewer incidents/accidents
- Reduced costs
- Reinforcement of operational goals of the organization

It is not designed to modify attitudes.

10)   Answer D.

CFR1910.178, Powered Industrial Trucks, requires anyone changing equipment or workplace location to meet the requirements outlined in the Refresher Training requirements (para 1910.178 (l)(4)). Only employees that are trained and authorized should operate industrial powered trucks.

11) Answer D.

According to the NSC, OJT or JIT is widely used because it allows the worker to produce during the training period. The primary instruction is the demonstration or demonstration-performance method of training.

12) Answer C.

There are two objectives to after-training testing. First, to see if the student has gained skill or knowledge in the subject area. Second, to assist the developer and instructor in evaluating the effectiveness of instruction. For example, if a significant percentage of students in an average class cannot perform up to the specifications outlined in the lesson plans, the instruction is simply not working. The problem could be atmosphere, instructional method, instruction techniques, instructor, training material, etc. Regardless, changes are in order. Effective training is a complex task in which evaluation of instruction is often overlooked. One thing that cannot be corrected by training is "poor worker attitude". This common complaint against the training staff is that worker attitudes haven't changed, but generally that is the responsibility of the supervisor.

13) Answer C.

Job performance is the most effective and final measure of any training program and training should be designed to correct skill deficiencies. Testing is highly recommended when effectiveness of training may be questioned.

14) Answer C.

The requirements of OSHA safety regulations for the safe use of ladders and stairs (Subpart X, Title 29 Code of Federal Regulations, Part 1926.1050 through 1926.1060) are explained in this discussion.

A stairway or ladder must be provided at all worker points of access where there is a break in elevation of 19 inches (48 cm) or more and no ramp, runway, embankment, or personnel hoist is provided.

When there is only one point of access between levels, it must be kept clear to permit free passage by workers. If free passage becomes restricted, a second point of access must be provided and used.

When there are more than two points of access between levels, at least one point of access must be kept clear.

All stairway and ladder fall protection systems required by these rules must be installed and all duties required by the stairway and ladder rules must be performed before employees begin work that requires them to use stairways or ladders and their respective fall protection systems.

15)   Answer B.

According to the OSHA Hazard Communication Standard (29 CFR 1926.59) employers shall provide employees with information and training on hazardous chemicals in their work area: at time of initial assignment; if transferred to a new assignment with new chemical hazards; or when a new chemical hazard is introduced into the work place.

16)   Answer C.

First a situation must be determined to be appropriate for the use of an extension cord. Then the power requirements of the tool (in amps) must be determined to match up the proper wire gauge and length of extension cord. Using an undersized extension cord can result in fire and electrical   hazards.

(NIOSH, 2009) NIOSH Publication No. 2009-113: Electrical Safety: Safety and Health for Electrical Trades Student Manual. Retrieved, NIOSH Publications and   Products

17)   Answer B.

Compressed gas cylinders in storage must be separated from other combustible material by a barrier that is non-combustible, has a 30 minute fire rating and is at least 5 feet high.

18)   Answer A.

1910.132(f)(1)

The employer shall provide training to each employee who is required by this section to use PPE. Each such employee shall be trained to know at least the following:

- When PPE is necessary

- What PPE is necessary
- How to properly don, doff, adjust, and wear PPE
- Limitations of PPE
- Proper care, maintenance, useful life and disposal of PPE

1910.132(f)(2)

Each affected employee shall demonstrate an understanding of the training specified in paragraph (f)(1) of this section, and the ability to use PPE properly, before being allowed to perform work requiring the use of PPE.

19)   Answer D.

The oxygen levels in confined space can decrease for many reasons, some not readily apparent to the person about to make entry. For example, the oxygen levels could decrease due to the nature of operations being conducted i.e.; welding, cutting, brazing etc. Certain chemical reactions (rusting) can cause an oxygen shortage or bacterial action (fermentation) can reduce the oxygen levels. *Ventilation* would not reduce the oxygen level, although it would aid in the mixing process.

20)   Answer A.

Supervisors are in the best position to provide realistic and effective training for industrial workers. They have detailed knowledge of work processes and control workflow.

21)   The best selection is answer D because:

The bottom line in any training or education effort is to provide a message that will be understood and acted on by the workers.

22)   Answer C.

A lesson plan is designed to insure the instructor:

- Presents material in the proper order
- Does not omit essential material
- Conducts training on proper timetable
- Places proper emphasis on items to be covered

- Provides for student participation
- Has confidence in presentation

23)   Answer A.

According to the NSC, communications is defined as "sharing information and/or ideas with others and being understood".

24)   Answer A.

According to the NSC, although statistical data differ, it is generally agreed that new employees are significantly more prone to work-related accidents.

25)   Answer C.

Face-to-face individual two-way communications are the best way to convey messages on the job.

Self-Assessment Quiz 6 Questions

1). Once a chemical has been classified, the hazard(s) must be communicated to target audiences. The exhibited pictogram represents which hazard class?

    A) Carcinogen.
    B) Irritant.
    C) Acute toxicity.
    D) Environmental toxicity.

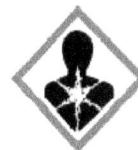

2). Safety training documentation should include all the following **EXCEPT**?

    A) Student's name
    B) Student's Social Security number
    C) Name and address of training provider
    D) Statement that student has successfully completed course

3). Industrial activities can generate considerable waste. Which of the following is **MOST** accurate?

    A) Hazardous waste must be diluted before disposal.
    B) All solid waste can be disposed of in the dumpsters provided at a workplace.
    C) Waste must be disposed of in accordance with local, state and federal regulations.
    D) All industrial solid wastes can be sent to special landfills.

4). When transiting the production area, a supervisor spots a safety hazard in a different department that presents imminent danger to contracted workers in the area. His/her first action should be to:

    A) Shut down production line and file a report.
    B) Bring the issue up in the next meeting.
    C) Post a lock-out/tag-out sign until hazard is corrected.
    D) Stop the work and notify area supervisor to get hazard corrected.\

5). When advising on decisions about workplace safety, the STS should:

    A) Always seek an outside opinion.
    B) Consult the local ASSE chapter for guidance when needed.
    C) Make biased independent decisions in all situations.
    D) Limit their advice and recommendation to those areas in which they have knowledge.

6). An employee, without eye protection, is observed installing parts at a bench. This is not a hazardous operation, but it is a posted "eye protection" area. Which of the following is the **BEST** course of action?

    A) Contact supervisor and discuss the situation.
    B) Test the new supervisor's skills by letting him handle the situation.
    C) Confront employee and determine why eye protection is not being used.
    D) Note discrepancy, but do not discuss it until the out brief when the CEO and supervisor are both present.

7). An object that connects a piece of electrical equipment to earth or some conducting body that serves in place of earth is a_____. It also serves to complete the electrical circuit and prevent the hazard to electrical shock caused by defective equipment, possibly causing death or serious injury.

    A) Bond.
    B) Ground.
    C) Metal frame.
    D) Double-insulation.

8). What is the definition of the management term "span of control"?

    A) The breadth of a manager's expertise.
    B) The number of subordinates a manager can supervise.
    C) The number of projects a manager can supervise.
    D) The number of organizations a manager can supervise.

9). When encountering unknown chemicals or potential asbestos-containing materials, what is the **FIRST** action a supervisor should do?

    A) Call an Industrial Hygienist.
    B) Stop work and have crew leave area.
    C) Call the company safety officer.
    D) Keep working until workers show signs and symptoms of exposure.

10). A CSP and licensed professional engineer asks a supervisor to informally review a series of fall protection plans for a warehouse construction project. The supervisor has adequately reviewed these types of plans for years, although without an engineering degree or formal fall protection system design education. Which statement most represents a reasonable interpretation of the STS Code of Ethics?

    A) A STS is qualified by exam to and permitted to approve employer safety programs.
    B) A STS is permitted to participate in a review of any construction related activity.
    C) The STS Code of Ethics permits only licensed professional engineers to determine whether other safety professionals have qualifications for reviewing their work.
    D) The STS Code of Ethics permits STSs to engage in work when they are qualified by experience in the specific technical fields involved, as well as by education.

11). A team member is working outside in 32°F cold weather. You see the person fall from a 12-foot step ladder and is lying unconscious. After sending someone for help, which best describes the **BEST** course of action?

    A) Verify the area is safe, adjust the injured person's head to ensure the worker is breathing.
    B) Verify the area is safe, do not move the injured person; check if the injured worker is breathing and assess for other injuries.
    C) Verify the area is safe, carefully move the injured person inside.
    D) Verify the area is safe, treat the person for shock and move the worker out of the cold and provide warm fluids.

12). All instruction manuals & operating procedure books for new equipment have been read by the STS. Upon completion of reading, what should be done with them?

    A) Communicate the information to the affected workers.
    B) Give them to the safety officer.
    C) Put them on the job site, and have workers go over them before starting work.
    D) Use them as a guide to develop a JSA

13). Trenches with a depth of 4 feet or greater must have a safe means of entry and egress and be inspected:

    A) Daily prior to start of work in trench.
    B) Prior to a rain storm.
    C) Once during a work shift.
    D) Post trench closure.

14). The one function that will always be filled at every emergency incident, regardless of size is the?

    A) Operations commander.
    B) Incident commander.
    C) Emergency Action coordinator.
    D) Medical staff.

15). Shipping hazardous waste requires an accompanying:

    A) Hazardous waste manifest.
    B) Safety data sheet (SDS).
    C) Chemical inventory if generated by a specified hazardous process.
    D) Hazardous waste list if generated in large quantities.

16). When impossible to interview people at the accident site, what is the next best location to interview a witness?

    A) Employee break room.
    B) Private conference room.
    C) Human resource office.
    D) Supervisor's office.

17). Safety training is best delivered by:

    A) An OSHA Compliance officer.
    B) The front-line supervisor.
    C) A contracted trainer.
    D) Co-workers.

18). To protect a crew on a scaffold near a busy roadway, a work zone barricade is designed for:

    A) Obstruction to deter pedestrians.
    B) Obstruction to warn pedestrians and vehicles.
    C) Obstruction to deter passage of vehicles and pedestrians.
    D) Obstruction to warn oncoming traffic.

19). Removing shoring from a trench must be performed:

    A) Top to bottom.
    B) Bottom to top.
    C) Middle down, then middle up.
    D) Any sequence determined best by supervisor.

20). Fire extinguishing equipment required for normal trash, such as paper or wood is:

    A) Class A ordinary combustibles extinguisher.
    B) Class B flammable liquid extinguisher.
    C) Class C electrical equipment fire extinguisher.
    D) Class K or F grease or cooking oil extinguisher.

21). Eye protection required for workers exposed to welding operations or individuals observing welding operations includes?

    A) Safety glasses.
    B) Goggles with filters.
    C) Flame proof screens or goggles.
    D) No protections required.

22). Development of emergency plans begins with:

    A) Conducting a basic risk assessment.
    B) Determining the location of emergency response resources
    C) Contacting the local fire department.
    D) Defining action plans that will be allowed by employees.

23). Guidelines for cleaning up a minor spill of flammable or combustible material include all **EXCEPT**?

    A) Immediately notify regulatory agencies of spill.
    B) Isolate spill site from non-required personnel.
    C) Block off spill area to prevent access.
    D) Remove electric hazards, incompatible chemicals or wastes, physical hazards and sources of ignition.

24). The rate of heat loss from exposed skin caused by wind and cold is defined as?

    A) Work temperature.
    B) Wind chill.
    C) Heat loss factor.
    D) Radiation decay.

25). Which activity is designed to verify if the management system is working, the emergency management administrative function is adequate and all lines of communication are operating?

    A) Dry run session.
    B) Practice session.
    C) Sandbox exercise.
    D) Tabletop exercise.

Self-Assessment Quiz 6 Answers

1) Answer A.

The GHS symbols have been incorporated into pictograms for use on the GHS label. Pictograms include the harmonized hazard symbols plus other graphic elements, such as borders, background patterns or colors which are intended to convey specific information. For transport, pictograms will have the background, symbol and colors currently used in the UN Recommendations on the Transport of Dangerous Goods, Model Regulations. For other sectors, pictograms will have a black symbol on a white background with a red diamond frame. A black frame may be used for shipments within one country. Where a transport pictogram appears, the GHS pictogram for the same hazard should not appear.

GHS Pictograms and Hazard Classes		
• Oxidizers	• Flammables • Self Reactives • Pyrophorics • Self-Heating • Emits Flammable Gas • Organic Peroxides	• Explosives • Self Reactives • Organic Peroxides
• Acute toxicity (severe)	• Corrosives	• Gases Under Pressure
• Carcinogen • Respiratory Sensitizer • Reproductive Toxicity • Target Organ Toxicity • Mutagenicity • Aspiration Toxicity	• Environmental Toxicity	• Irritant • Dermal Sensitizer • Acute toxicity (harmful) • Narcotic Effects • Respiratory Tract Irritation

2)   Answer B.

Written documentation should be provided to each student who satisfactorily completes the training course. The documentation should include:

- Student's name
- Course title
- Course date
- Statement that student has successfully completed the course
- Name and address of training provider
- An individual identification number for certificate
- List of levels of personal protective equipment used by student to complete the course.

This documentation may include a certificate and an appropriate wallet sized laminated card with a photograph of the student and above information. When such course certificate cards are used, the individual identification number for the training certificate should be shown on the card.

Recordkeeping. Training providers should maintain records listing dates courses were presented, the names of individual course attendees, names of those students successfully completing each course, and number of training certificates issued to each successful student. These records should be maintained for a minimum of five years after the date an individual participated in a training program offered by the training provider. These records should be available and provided upon the student's request or as mandated by law.

3)   Answer C.

Most of waste generated by construction activities is non-hazardous solid waste and can be disposed of in appropriately licensed landfills. Hazardous waste must be identified and properly stored, transported and disposed of. Hazardous waste cannot be disposed of in most landfills. No federal requirements exist for all large construction projects to recycle construction debris.

4)   Answer D.

If workers are in eminent danger, the best is to stop the work and notify the direct supervisor. The person to correct the hazard should be the individual with the most area knowledge, that is, the area supervisor.

5)   Answer D.

This can be a difficult question, but the BEST answer of those listed is to only make recommendations if certain that the result will ensure a safer work area. Making recommendations about unskilled areas has the potential to be incorrect.

6)   Answer A.

The first action should be to contact the supervisor who has control of the workplace and discuss the infraction. Further action may include some of the other solutions presented in the above options.

7)   Answer B.

The term "ground" refers to a conductive body, usually the earth. "Grounding" a tool or electrical system means intentionally creating a low-resistance path to the earth. When properly done, current from a short or from lightning follows this path, thus preventing the buildup of voltages that would otherwise result in electrical shock, injury and even death.

8)   Answer B.

The well-known principle of "span of control" is defined as recognition that a manager cannot effectively supervise more than half a dozen subordinate managers.

9)   Answer B.

Stop work and have the crew leave the area; then notify direct manager. Industrial hygienists are commonly used to determine chemical exposure.

10)   Answer D.

The second standard in the STS Code of Ethics states that a STS shall "Perform safety responsibilities and assignments only in areas of their competence." Competence can be achieved through formal training, on-the-job training and experience.

11)   Answer B.

The general recommendation is not to move the injured worker; victims of falls are at risk for spinal injuries. Moving the injured worker could result in their death or permanent paralysis. Always ensure the area is safe for responders before assisting someone else.

12)   Answer A.

Reviewing the manual with workers is the next step.

13)   Answer A.

According to 29 CFR 1926, Subpart P. Excavations, Inspections shall be made by a competent person and should be documented. The following guide specifies the frequency and conditions requiring inspections:

- Daily and before the start of each shift
- As dictated by the work being done in the trench
- After every rainstorm
- After other events that could increase hazards, e.g. snowstorm, windstorm, thaw, earthquake, etc.
- When fissures, tension cracks, sloughing, undercutting, water seepage, bulging at the bottom, or other similar conditions occur
- When there is a change in size, location, or placement of spoil pile and
- When there is any indication of change or movement in adjacent structures

14)   Answer B.

According to the NSC, the one function that will always be filled at every incident, regardless of size, is the Incident Commander. For small operations, the most likely incident commander will be the Fire Chief, due to greater experience, more equipment involved and more training than facility staff.

15)   Answer A.

This section does not apply to: Any hazardous waste as such term is defined by the Solid Waste Disposal Act, as amended by the Resource Conservation and Recovery Act of 1976, as amended (42 U.S.C. 6901 et seq.), when subject to regulations issued under that Act by the Environmental Protection Agency.

16)   Answer B.

The best place to interview a witness during an accident investigation is the accident site. If this is not possible, a private location that will not intimidate, inhibit or distract the witness is preferred. A worker's or supervisor's office may be intimidating.

17)   Answer B.

Safety training is best delivered by the front-line supervisor.

18)   The best selection is answer C because:

As defined by 29 CFR 1926.203, a barricade is an obstruction to deter the passage of vehicles and pedestrians.

19)   Answer B.

1926.652(e)(1)(v): Removal shall begin at, and progress from, the bottom of the excavation. Members shall be released slowly so as to note any indication of possible failure of the remaining members of the structure or possible cave-in of the sides of the excavation.

20)   Answer A.

1910.252(a)(2)(ii): Fire extinguishers. Suitable fire extinguishing equipment shall be maintained in a state of readiness for instant use. Such equipment may consist of pails of water, buckets of sand, hose or portable extinguishers depending upon the nature and quantity of the combustible material exposed.

Six Types of Fire Extinguishers

1. Class A – Wood, Paper, Plastics
2. Class AB – Wood, Paper and Flammable Liquid
3. Class BC (flammable liquid and electrical)
4. Class ABC Multipurpose
5. Class D – Metal Fires
6. Class K or F – Kitchen Fire

CLASSES OF FIRES	TYPES OF FIRES	PICTURE SYMBOL
A	Wood, paper, cloth, trash & other ordinary materials.	
B	Gasoline, oil, paint and other flammable liquids.	
C	May be used on fires involving live electrical equipment without danger to the operator.	
D	Combustible metals and combustible metal alloys.	
K	Cooking media (Vegetable or Animal Oils and Fats)	

21) Answer C.

As per OSHA 1910.252, Helmets or hand shields shall be used during all arc welding or arc cutting operations, excluding submerged arc welding. Helpers or attendants shall be provided with proper eye protection. Protection from arc welding rays. Where the work permits, the welder should be enclosed in an individual booth painted with a finish of low reflectivity such as zinc oxide (an important factor for absorbing ultraviolet radiations) and lamp black, or shall be enclosed with noncombustible screens similarly painted. Booths and screens shall permit circulation of air at floor level. Workers or other persons adjacent to the welding areas shall be protected from the rays by noncombustible or flameproof screens or shields or shall be required to wear appropriate goggles.

22) Answer A.

Development of emergency plans begins with conducting a basic risk assessment. The first step is to identify the types of emergencies or disasters that a company is at risk for and then to evaluate the potential harm to people, property and operations to help prioritize the risks. An organization in Florida will want to spend considerable time planning for a hurricane, a facility in the Midwest should plan for Tornados, while a company in northern California should plan for an earthquake.

23) Answer A.

You are not required to notify OSHA for a minor spill;, however, you need to isolate the area for clean-up and remove all hazards, including ignition sources, especially if the spill is flammable.

24) Answer B.

The wind chill temperature is how cold people and animals feel when outside. Wind chill is based on rate of heat loss from exposed skin caused by wind and cold. As the wind increases, it draws heat from the body, driving down skin temperature and eventually internal body temperature. Therefore, wind makes it FEEL much colder. If the temperature is 0 degrees Fahrenheit and the wind is blowing at 15 mph, the wind chill is 19 degrees Fahrenheit. At this wind chill temperature, exposed skin can freeze in 30 minutes.

Wind Chill Factor is caused by increased wind speeds which accelerate heat loss from exposed skin. No specific rules exist for determining when wind chill becomes dangerous. As a general rule, the threshold for potentially dangerous wind chill conditions is about 20°F. Wind chill factor is the major concern when exposing workers to the elements.

25) Answer D.

A tabletop exercise (TTX) involves senior staff, elected or appointed officials, or other key personnel in an informal group discussion centered on a hypothetical scenario.

In a TTX, participants:

- Identify strengths and shortfalls.
- Enhance understanding of new concepts.
- Seek to change existing attitudes and perspectives.

Conduct Characteristics

- Requires an experienced facilitator.
- In-depth discussion.
- Slow-paced problem solving.

The purpose of a TTX is to test existing plans, policies, or procedures without incurring the costs associated with deploying resources. A TTX also allows participants to thoroughly work through a problem without feeling as much pressure as they would in an operations-based exercise. (FEMA 2016)

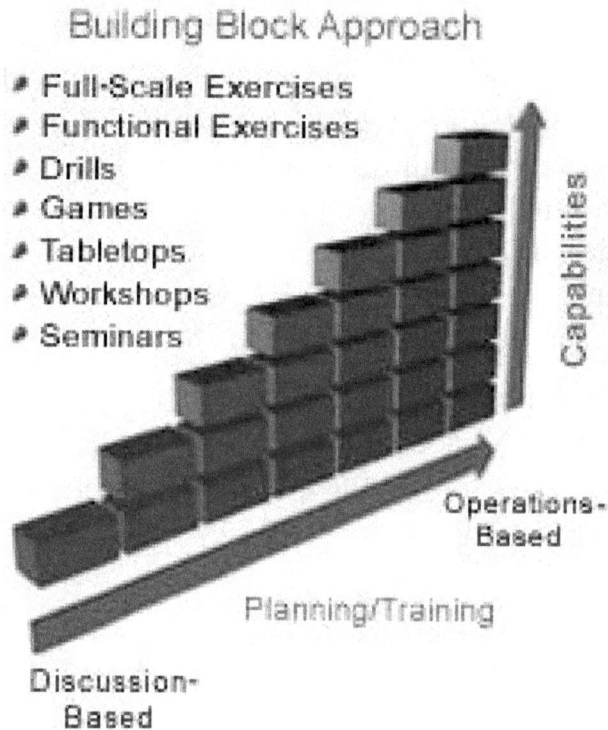

STS Self-Assessment Practice Exam

Given 135 minutes, determine the number of questions answered correctly.

Self-Assessment Practice Exam Questions

1).   Which of the following **best** describes the Threshold Limit Value (TLV)?

   A) The amount of hazardous chemical exposure to which a worker can be exposed.
   B) The number of physical hazards to which a worker can be exposed.
   C) The amount of hazardous chemicals in work area.
   D) The required information on a container label.

2).   Respirator users must be trained, medically cleared, and

   A) Assigned a personal respirator.
   B) Purchase their own respirator.
   C) Provided a new respirator daily.
   D) Fit tested.

3).   Your crew enters an area and finds used disposable respirators on the floor from a previous work crew. Your company has a respirator program and as the supervisor you should:

   A) Begin work and assume the previous hazard has been removed.
   B) Put all workers in the respirators left by the previous crew.
   C) Determine the reason for the previous crew's usage of the respirator and appropriately protect the crew from those hazards.
   D) Begin work and write a report to the contracting employer.

4).   Your company does not have a respirator program. The Supervisor and crew arrive on site to begin work outside. About 20 meters (60 feet) upwind from the work area, a welding crew is still working in respirators. The welding crew supervisor said they would be finished in 20 minutes. The supervisor should:

   A) Begin work.
   B) Put the crew in respirators and begin work.
   C) Wait the 20 min for the welders to complete their work.
   D) Have the welding crew supervisor suspend operations until your crew is finished.

5). Work in a confined space monitor reads 15% oxygen. The workers should:

    A) Evacuate, the space is oxygen enriched.
    B) Continue working.
    C) Evacuate, the space is oxygen deficient.
    D) Put the workers in air purifying respirators.

6). On a jobsite, which of the following is **most correct** concerning Safety Data Sheets (SDS) accessibility?

    A) The supervisor or crew leader must have access and can provide a copy to the workers.
    B) Provide a copy for each worker for each chemical.
    C) Copies of SDS should be filed with the local fire department.
    D) SDS are provided to the workers by OSHA.

7). When workers enter a permit required confined space with hazardous conditions, who must have continuous communication with the entrants?

    A) One attendant per entrant.
    B) A rescue team available within 30 seconds.
    C) Entry supervisor.
    D) Attendant(s).

8). Which of the following terms **best** describes when to dispose of a respirator?

    A) Service life.
    B) Protection factor.
    C) Air purifying.
    D) Fit test.

9). Which is the **most appropriate** measurement of individual safety performance?

    A) Recognize workers for reporting hazards and correcting them.
    B) Group performing thus far without injuries.
    C) No safety discipline in the past year.
    D) Crew completes entire job without a recordable injury.

10). The Superintendent asks a STSC to evaluate the injury records for a 1 Million-Man-Hours-With-No-Lost-Time Accident Award. Upon review, the STS discovers that a case involving 3 days away from work was not categorized correctly. The STSC should:

    A) Report the misclassification to the site superintendent.
    B) Allow recognition to continue.
    C) Notify the federal authorities.
    D) Do not issue the award.

11). Which of following **most** relates to the 1st standard of the STS code of ethics?

    A) Perform safety responsibilities and assignments only in areas of their competence.
    B) Hold paramount the safety and health of people and the protection of property and environment in performance of safety responsibilities.
    C) Issue objective and truthful statements to employers, clients or appropriate authorities.
    D) Act in matters related to safety responsibilities for employers or clients as faithful agents.

12). A Foreman requests that the STSC conduct samples on the dust from a grinding operation. The STSC has no experience with collecting samples. The STSC should:

    A) Notify superintendent that STS is not qualified and recommend the company gets a qualified person to collect samples.
    B) Read up on specific materials and perform sampling.
    C) Recommend proceeding with job without sampling.
    D) Put crew in respirators.

13). The Site Manager requests that STSC go to training to enhance skills related to safety on the job. The STSC should:

    A) Decline the training if possessing all necessary skills.
    B) Attend first half of training to determine if relevant.
    C) Go to training, as per STS Code of Ethics requiring continuous professional development.
    D) Make verbal commitment, but do not attend training.

14). When is training **least appropriate?**

    A) At the beginning of shift.
    B) After an incident.
    C) After a recordable injury.
    D) At end of work shift.

15). Who is **most responsible** for ensuring a union worker follows safety rules?

    A) Union representative.
    B) Site manager.
    C) Union representative on safety committee.
    D) Line supervisor.

16). Gas cylinders' safety valve covers must be in place always **except** when:

    A) In transport.
    B) On cart.
    C) In use.
    D) In job trailer.

17). Organizational goals and objectives should meet targets that are:

    A) Measurable, actionable, rigorous, specific, open-ended.
    B) Special, measurable, actionable, opportunistic, timed.
    C) Specific, measurable, actionable, realistic, time-bound.
    D) Subjective, actionable, regulatory, measureable, time-bound.

18). A group of managers and supervisors are reviewing the emergency planning and response. Communications and procedures were tested, but no equipment was mobilized nor hands on performed. This type of exercise is called a:

    A) Table top.
    B) Functional.
    C) Tactical drill.
    D) Full-scale scenario.

19). The **best** selection of people for a safety committee is:

A) Upper and mid-level manager.
B) Supervisors and line workers.
C) Company owners and shareholders.
D) Contractors and government officials.

20). Who is primarily responsible for enforcing safety rules:

A) Supervisor.
B) Crew members.
C) Project manager.
D) Government regulators.

21). An STSC goes into an area with several unsafe conditions involving different subcontractors. The STSC should:

A) Allow work to continue.
B) Write a report to the project manager.
C) Submit a report to regulatory agencies.
D) Stop work and discuss with department supervisors.

22). Your work crew notices contractor employees in an area they are not normally working in. The **best** action as a supervisor is to:

A) Report the issue to the facilities manager.
B) Suspend operations and ask the contractor employees what they are doing.
C) Continue work and observe contractor employees for safety violations.
D) Assume they are supposed to be there and continue work.

23). Workplace hazard information should be communicated in:

A) A language and symbols that workers and management understand.
B) English.
C) The language of the workers.
D) All languages.

24). A container used for oily rags must be:

    A) Placed in a plastic container.
    B) Placed in an approved metal can and covered with lid.
    C) Placed in a metal can.
    D) Placed in a labeled bucket.

25). If there are hazardous waste organic solvents from an operation, the supervisor should:

    A) Notify company environmental manager and ask what to do with the materials.
    B) Let evaporate and place in trash.
    C) Place in trash and cover with other construction debris.
    D) Leave on site for contractor cleanup crews.

26). A hearing conservation program is triggered when sound levels reach the 85-decibel action limit. What is the **primary** purpose of annual audio metric testing?

    A) To establish the appropriate noise reduction rating (NRR).
    B) To prevent occupational hearing loss.
    C) To comply with safety regulations.
    D) To monitor workers' hearing health.

27). The **primary** purpose of a safety meeting is:

    A) Provide discipline to workers not following safety rules.
    B) Inform workers of job specific hazards.
    C) Satisfy government regulations.
    D) Document meeting attendance.

28). In behavior-based safety programs, Antecedent-Behavior-Consequence Analysis is often used to evaluate safety performance. In terms of consequences, the **strongest** and **most powerful** influencers are:

    A) Soon, Uncertain, and Negative.
    B) Latent, Uncertain, and Positive.
    C) Soon, Certain, and Positive.
    D) Latent, Certain, and Negative.

29). Scissor and aerial lifts are considered:

   A) Stationary scaffolds.
   B) Mobile scaffolds.
   C) Powered industrial trucks.
   D) Fixed work platforms.

30). Where should the employee attach their safety lanyard to an anchor point?

   A) The attachment of the body harness D ring must be in the center of the wearer's back, near the shoulder level, or above the head.
   B) The safety lanyard should be attached to the building's structural supports.
   C) The safety lanyard should be attached to any convenient point capable of supporting the employee's weight.
   D) Tie offs are not recommended so the employee can escape the basket in the event of a boom failure.

31). An example a human factor contributing to an incident is:

   A) Operator fatigue.
   B) Procedures not clearly written.
   C) Equipment malfunction.
   D) Machinery unguarded.

32). In the accident investigation context, a safety procedure is an example of

   A) A management system.
   B) An event.
   C) A direct cause.
   D) Causation.

33). By how much will the safe working load (SWL) lifting capacity of the sling be reduced when each leg's angle to the vertical is a 45° angle?
   A) 25%.
   B) 60%.
   C) 30%.
   D) 75%.

34). New hire employees should be trained:

    A) Initially and before exposed to the hazards on the job site.
    B) After 30 days.
    C) After 60 days.
    D) During the first week.

35). All machines consist of these fundamental areas:

    A) The point of operation, the power transmission device, and the operating controls.
    B) The point of operation, the power switch, and the safety guards.
    C) The cutting surface, the power switch, and the operating controls.
    D) The cutting surface, the power transmission device, and the machine guarding.

36). Heat stress management is **best** accomplished by:

    A) Assuring that only persons that have passed stress tests by a health care professional.
    B) Provide salt tablets and electrolyte drinks to allow workers to perform full duties.
    C) Monitor workers, provide hydration and food when worker activity decreases.
    D) Training for supervisors and workers to prevent, recognize, and treat heat-related illness.

37). A ladder must extend above the working surface:

    A) 0.3 meter (1 foot).
    B) 1 meter (3 feet).
    C) 2 meters (6 feet).
    D) 3 meters (9 feet).

38). Which of the following **best** describes the cumulative trauma disorder (CTD) carpal tunnel syndrome?

    A) Elbow and shoulder swelling and inflammation.
    B) Inflammation of the channel in the wrist.
    C) Raynaud's syndrome of the hand and wrist.
    D) White finger.

39). The **MOST** important information on a Safety Data Sheet (SDS) is:

A) The name and structure of chemical equations.
B) The emergency procedures and first aid for chemical exposure.
C) The environmental disposal procedures.
D) The Inert ingredients of a hazardous mixture.

40). Matching the task to the worker is the definition of:

A) Kinesiology.
B) Anthropometry.
C) Physiology.
D) Ergonomics.

41). Chemicals that cause permanent changes to an exposed worker's genetic material (DNA) are called:

A) Irritants.
B) Sensitizers.
C) Mutagens.
D) Teratogens.

42). The highest level of respiratory protection for entering an Immediately Dangerous to Life and Health (IDLH) workplace environment is:

A) Self-Contained Breathing Apparatus (SCBA).
B) Supplied Air Respirator (SAR).
C) Powered Air Purifying Respirator (PAPR).
D) Air Purifying Respirator (APR).

43). The point where the blade of a table saw engages the wood to be cut is called the:

A) Pinch point.
B) Shear point.
C) Hazardous operation.
D) Point of operation.

44). Hard hat usage is determined by types of overhead hazards and the presence of

    A) Solar heat load hazards.
    B) Fall hazards.
    C) Electrical hazards.
    D) Confined space hazards.

45). The **first** item to check before beginning crane operations is for:

    A) Rear swing radius.
    B) Overhead power lines.
    C) Barricade work zone.
    D) Load weight to be picked.

46). A heavy equipment operator must:

    A) Have a valid state driver's license.
    B) Be properly trained and authorized.
    C) Have worked on the site for at least a week.
    D) Be OSHA certified.

47). The **most important** consideration before lifting a load with a crane is to:

    A) Secure rear swing radius.
    B) Check load rating of the floor.
    C) Determine hand signals with operator.
    D) Know the crane capacity and weight of load.

48). The **primary** method for ensuring synthetic sling integrity is:

    A) Hourly, by equipment operator.
    B) Daily, pre-use visual inspections.
    C) Monthly visual inspection.
    D) Annually sling proof-testing.

49). What is the **best** course of action if supervisors witness an experienced worker not following safety rules?
    A) Stop work, correct the worker, follow company disciplinary procedures.
    B) Ignore and avoid confrontation.

C) Assume experienced worker knows how to safety perform task.
D) Speak to worker the next day.

50). When a new, inexperienced worker breaks a safety rule, the supervisor should:

A) Stop work, correct the worker.
B) Stop work, discipline worker.
C) Allow work to continue and have a meeting with worker at the shift end.
D) Report worker to site management.

51). People will model behavior that they view are beneficial; therefore, workers are **more likely** to follow rules when:

A) Contractors are seen bypassing rules.
B) The leadership demonstrates the importance of safety rules.
C) Workers are sometimes disciplined for breaking safety rules.
D) They see fellow workers punished when caught breaking rules.

52). What is the term used for protecting workers from exposure to blood and bodily fluids?

A) Disinfecting PPE.
B) Contamination control.
C) Exposure incident.
D) Universal precautions.

53). The **most important** item to verify when testing a flexible extension cord is:

A) Double insulation.
B) Proper ground.
C) Length and resistance.
D) Voltage capacity.

54). Which is the **best** definition of hazard?

A) A condition, set of circumstances, or inherent property that can cause injury, illness, or death.

B) An event in which a work-related injury, illness, or fatality occurred or could have occurred.

C) A set of interrelated elements that establish and support occupational safety and health objectives.

D) An estimate of the combination of the likelihood of an occurrence of a hazardous event or exposure, and the severity of the injury.

55). Risk is a combination of:

A) Frequency of episodes of an adverse event and probability of occurrence of the adverse event.

B) Probability that an adverse event will occur and consequences of the adverse event.

C) Probability that a hazardous condition exists and consequences of the hazard.

D) Exposure and consequences to a particular hazard.

56). The **best** solution to a hazard in the workplace is:

A) Barricade the hazard.

B) Eliminate the hazard.

C) Train affected workers on hazard.

D) Continue work and report hazard to controlling employer.

57). What is the **primary** function of a loss control system?

A) Assess risk, establish effective risk control measures, and elimination of risk.

B) Establish effective risk control measures for hazardous conditions, establish effective control measures, elimination of risk.

C) Identify hazardous conditions, assess their risks, and establish effective risk control measures.

D) Assure compliance with applicable regulatory requirements and eliminate residual risk.

58). Which of the following is the **best** description of an aerosol?

A) Suspension of liquid particles formed by condensation.

B) Suspension of liquid or solid particles dispersed in air.

C) Solid particle in air formed by condensation.

D) Particulate material in air.

59). When the noise level exceeds permissible limits, the use of PPE requires the employer to:

    A) See that cotton plugs are clean, and workers are trained to insert properly.

    B) Provide a standardized formed earplug that attenuates all noise levels to below 70 decibels.

    C) Ensure that everyone has had an audiometric exam and instruct employees to purchase hearing protection with the proper noise reduction rating (NRR).

    D) Provide at least two types of hearing protection with the proper noise reduction rating (NRR) and instruct employees on proper use/wearing.

60). After an accident, the priority is taking care of any injured persons. What should be the next priority?

    A) Secure the area.

    B) Make statements about the cause.

    C) Start interviewing people.

    D) Start your accident report.

61). What is **most important** for a worker to know before isolating a machine?

    A) Manufacturer of the machine.

    B) The specific energy isolation locations and devices.

    C) Lock out policy.

    D) OSHA lock out standard.

62). Who is the **best** person for insuring that workers are wearing the appropriate PPE?

    E) The Project Manager.

    F) The Supervisor.

    G) A Safety Person.

    H) An OSHA Officer.

63). On multi-employer work sites, what is the **best** method for one employer to inform the other employers about new Safety Data Sheets (SDS) for chemicals?

    A) Develop a system for the general contractor and subcontractors to share SDS.
    B) The general contractor is responsible.
    C) The superintendent should see that everyone is informed.
    D) Everyone should be responsible for their own.

64). Generally, system life cycle phases include:

    A) Concept, development, operation, disposal.
    B) Initiation, development, design, evaluation.
    C) Analysis, design, production, disposal.
    D) Concept, sustainment, reliability, disposal.

65). A key factor for implementing a good Safety Program involves:

    A) Getting employees motivated.
    B) Having a good training program.
    C) Getting foreman and supervisors involved.
    D) Cheaper insurance.

66). The company health and safety officer completed a Job Safety Analysis (JSA) for a supervisor's task and forwarded it to the field. Once JSA is received and reviewed, it is apparent that there are more hazards to the task than are listed on the JSA. What should you do?

    A) Send the JSA back to the health and safety officer and do not begin work on the task until the JSA has been revised to reflect status change of hazard.
    B) Read and understand hazards on JSA, make any corrections to it prior to use and send revisions back to the safety officer.
    C) Send the JSA back to the health and safety officer.
    D) Begin working on the task using the information listed on the JSA.

67). When interviewing a witness during an accident investigation, what is the **best** approach?

A) Interview witnesses one at a time.
B) Interviews should be conducted at the site.
C) Take notes or record the interview.
D) Interview witnesses together for a "big picture"

68). Which represents the **best** way to reduce at risk behaviors?
A) Enter the workers into a progressive discipline program.
B) Consistently applying positive reinforcement to appropriate behavior.
C) Implement a behavior-based safety program.
D) Wait until there is a serious injury and focus on lessons learned.

69). What is the **primary** purpose of accident investigation?

A) To establish fault.
B) To prevent recurrence based on similar causes.
C) To find the root cause.
D) To report accidents and near misses.

70). It is a generally accepted theory in accident prevention that the attitude of supervisors and managers can affect the actions of foreman and employees. Which of the following **best** describes that relationship?
A) Supervisor's attitudes have no effect on employees.
B) Supervisor's attitudes have little effect on employees.
C) Supervisor's attitude has a direct influence on employees.
D) Supervisor's attitudes have a direct influence, which cannot be changed.

71). Which of the following is the **most likely** explanation for a new hire that is not working safely after attending safety orientation?

A) Training objectives are different than work objectives.
B) Trainer did not present the information effectively.
C) Training objectives are the same as workplace rules.
D) Trainer followed the training outline

72). Why should supervisors discuss the results of safety inspections with their employees?

A) To give positive reinforcement for good work practice and discuss

hazards and corrective measures.
B) To determine disciplinary actions.
C) To find the root cause.
D) To report accidents and near misses.

73). The type of supervisor skill demonstrated through empathy, rephrasing and repeating is called:

A) Nonverbal communication.
B) Effective listening.
C) Observation reinforcement.
D) Immediate feedback.

74). Which of the following conditions is **least likely** to require the workers to wear a hard hat?

A) Around energized electrical lines.
B) Where the possibility of falling objects exists.
C) Around heavy equipment.
D) When overhead bump hazards are greater than 7 feet from the working surface.

75). What resource can **best** instruct supervisors on how to operate a tool safely?

A) The OSHA compliance officer.
B) The production manager.
C) The tool manufacturer instruction manual.
D) The site safety officer.

76). Which of the following is **not** a recognized form of PPE?

A) Back braces.
B) Hard hats.
C) Gloves.
D) Face shields.

77). Which is the **best** protection for pouring a caustic chemical:

A) Chemical splash goggles and face shield.
B) Goggles.
C) Face shield.

D) Safety glasses with side shields.

78). You notice a work team is not implementing new hazard controls that were recently changed in a Job Safety Analysis (JSA). Which represents the **best** approach to motivate the team to improve performance?

A) Enter the work team into the company progressive disciplinary process.
B) Provide an oral reprimand for failing to follow safety rules.
C) Send the work team back to the safety manager for retraining.
D) Communicate the change, remain in the area and observe.

79). Nausea, sweating and dizziness are symptoms of which of the following?

A) Heat exhaustion.
B) Heat stroke.
C) Heat stress.
D) Heat rash.

80). What are the three major exposure paths for chemical compounds to enter the body?

A) Nose, eyes and mouth.
B) Inhaled, skin contact, and swallowed.
C) Inhaled, through hands, and injected.
D) Absorption, adsorption and inhalation.

81). The bloodborne pathogen standard requires that people must be trained when cleaning up:

A) Human blood and body fluids.
B) Infectious waste.
C) Contaminated needles.
D) Construction debris waste.

82). An example of an energy isolation device is a:

A) Tagout system.
B) Push buttons.
C) Disconnect switch.
D) Selector switch.

83). Which of the following is considered to be the **primary** reason for accident investigation for Safety and Health reasons?

    A) To determine the facts surrounding the event.
    B) To establish who or what was at fault.
    C) To determine the obvious cause factors.
    D) To establish a baseline for further analysis.

84). Who has responsibility for safety at multiple-employer work sites?
    A) The direct employer.
    B) The construction manager.
    C) The client and the subcontractor.
    D) All employers and employees on the site.

85). When transporting, moving or storing compressed cylinders, what must be in place?

    A) Valve stems with gauge.
    B) Valve protection caps.
    C) Hoses with anti-flashback valves.
    D) Pressure regulators.

86). Emergency planning should be conducted:

    A) 30 days after work has begun.
    B) Prior to work beginning at the site.
    C) During the first week on site.
    D) Immediately following an emergency.

87). Emergency eyewash stations should be able to flush the eyes for a minimum of:

    A) 10 minutes.
    B) 15 minutes.
    C) 25 minutes.
    D) 30 minutes.

88). The **final** step in an incident investigation process is:

    A) Interview witnesses.
    B) Determine the corrective actions.
    C) Ensure corrective items are initiated.

D) Train the workers.

89). At **minimum**, documentation of training includes student name, topic outline, objectives, date and:

A) Trainer name and qualifications.
B) Multi-media presentation.
C) Pre- and post-test scores.
D) Literacy equivalency.

90). After safety training is completed, there are many ways to encourage workplace safety performance. The **best** examples of leadership include:

A) Setting a good example, encouraging safe behavior, follow up on complaints and hazard reports.
B) Setting a good example, strictly enforcing all safety requirements, follow up on complaints and hazard reports.
C) Encouraging safe behavior, require persons that report problems to fix them, setting a good example.
D) Getting worker to clearly document their safety concerns, strictly enforcing all safety requirements, performing surprise checks of equipment.

91). The **primary** purpose of worker safety training and education programs is:

A) To prepare for testing.
B) To meet regulatory requirements.
C) To minimize insurance premiums.
D) To impart knowledge, skill and ability.

92). The **most important** element of safety management system comes from:

A) Demonstrated management leadership.
B) Employee compliance with work rules.
C) Written policy and programs.
D) Safety inspections identifying workplace hazards.

93). A first responder trained supervisor sees sparks and observes a worker fall to the ground while using power tools. The supervisor should:

A) Secure sources of electricity, send someone to call for emergency services, assess the worker's injuries, care for the victim within the limits of responders training.

B) Immediately send someone to call for emergency services, check the victim for respirations and pulse, start CPR and give them oxygen.

C) Call for emergency services, check the victim for respirations and pulse, and start CPR or apply the AED.

D) Check the victim for respirations and a pulse, send someone to call for emergency services, remove the victim from the work area and start First Aid and CPR as appropriate.

94). A worker reports that a ladder has a split up the side rail, the **best** action is to:

A) Continue using and replace at end of week.

B) Use a 2x4 board as a splint for side rail.

C) Remove from service, tag it, and inform crew not to use.

D) Secure with duct tape and continue usage.

95). Electrical equipment will continue to operate if:

A) Neutral wire is disconnected.

B) Current carrying wire is disconnected.

C) Ground wire is disconnected.

D) Current carrying wire is shorted to ground.

96). A device that prevents the back-flow mixing of oxygen and acetylene is called a:

A) Pressure relief.

B) Check valve.

C) Screw plug.

D) Vent terminus.

97). What is the order of hazard hierarchy control methods from **most effective** to **least effective?**

   A.) Substitution, elimination, engineering controls, warnings, administrative controls, personal protective equipment.
   B.) Elimination, engineering controls, substitution, administrative controls, warnings, personal protective equipment.
   C.) Engineering controls, Elimination, substitution, administrative controls, warnings, personal protective equipment.
   D.) Elimination, substitution, engineering controls, warnings, administrative controls, personal protective equipment.

98). The **best** computer workstation design adjusts to the worker so that:

   A) Arms hang loose, elbows at 90 angles, forearms inline, and wrists supported.
   B) Arms are rigid, elbows above a 90 angle, forearms raised, and wrists slightly bent.
   C) Forearms straight, shoulders relaxed, knees below the hips, and feet slightly backward.
   D) Shoulders rigid, arms parallel to the floor, knees aligned with hips, and feet slightly forward.

99). The **most effective** safety and health activities:

   A) Are incorporated into operations of the business and are integrated in already functioning activities, whenever possible.
   B) Are supported by trained and qualified safety professionals and are accomplished in a manner to guarantee independence from already existing activities, which may be performed incorrectly.
   C) Provide a substantial check and balance to already existing activities, when performed independently by a third party.
   D) Will disrupt business activities and cause trades people to delay completion of their work.

100). An employee who isolates the energy from machines or equipment to perform servicing or maintenance on that machine or equipment is considered a(n):

A) Affected employee.
B) Authorized attendant.
C) Qualified person.
D) Authorized employee.

Self-Assessment Practice Exam Answers

1)   Answer A.

The TLV lists the exposure amount for chemicals

2)   The best selection is answer D because:

Respirator users must be trained, medically cleared, and properly fit-tested.

3)   Answer C.

Hazard determination is the first step in protecting workers. Determining the reason for the previous crew's respirator usage will allow supervisors to appropriately protect the crew from those hazards.

4)   Answer C.

In this case it would be best just to wait 20 minutes and allow other crew to complete their work.

5)   Answer C.

A confined space with less than 19.5% oxygen is considered oxygen deficient and the crew must be evacuated of supplied air if not provided or if continuous ventilation verifies oxygen level is between 19.5% and 23.5%.

6)   Answer A.

SDS must be accessible to employees and their representatives in a reasonable amount of time. The supervisor must have access to share with employees.

7)   Answer D.

Workers in a confined space with hazardous conditions should be provided with attendant(s) with for continuous visual communication with all entrants.

8)   Answer A.

The employer must determine the end of service life (ESL) for a respirator, based on chemical exposure and manufacturer's recommendations.

9)   Answer A.

Positive reinforcement is the best motivator. Recognizing workers for reporting hazards and correcting them is a positive individual metric for safety performance.

10)   Answer A.

The best solution in this example is to communicate the discrepancy with the site superintendent.

11)   The best selection is answer B because:

"Hold paramount the safety and health of people, and protection of property and the environment in performance of safety responsibilities" is the first standard listed in the STS code of ethics.

12)   Answer A.

The STS code of ethics states that an STS should perform safety responsibilities and assignments **only** in areas of their competence.

13)   Answer C.

An STS should always look for opportunities to improve one's professional skill set.

14)   Answer D.

Training is least effective and appropriate at the end of the work shift.

15)   Answer D.

Line supervisor is the most able and responsible for ensuring workers follow safety rules. It is the employer's responsibility to determine and enforce the rules.

16)   Answer C.

Gas cylinders safety valve covers must be on at all times, except when in use.

17)   Answer C.

Objectives should meet targets, ANSI Z-10 using the example of "SMART" criteria:

- Specific—Clearly defined desired outcome
- Measurable—Concrete metric for success
- Actionable—Written as a concrete action plan
- Realistic—Practical in its scope
- Time-bounded—A specific timeframe is set

When choosing an appropriate organizational model, a manager should understand that there are multiple arrangements that will produce the best result with minimum difficulty in the situation in which the organization operates. Given individual discretion and the fact that some configurations appear to influence employee performance and satisfaction, managers should consider carefully the behavioral implications when making decisions.

18)   Answer A.

A table top exercise is the technique that best describes this type of emergency planning activity.

19)   Answer B.

A Safety committee should be a good representation of the organization. Supervisors and workers are critical members of a safety committee.

20) Answer A.

The supervisor generally has the primary responsibility for enforcing safety rules.

21) Answer D.

The best approach is to do the work and discuss the situation with supervisors from all contractors involved with the operation in question.

22) Answer B.

A supervisor must stop and investigate suspicious activity from other contracting crews.

23) Answer A.

Hazardous chemical labels should be written in a language and symbols so that workers and management can read and identify hazards.

24) The best selection is answer B because:

Oily rags should be placed in an approved metal can and covered with lid.

25) Answer A.

A supervisor should notify company environmental manager and determine what to do with hazardous materials waste.

26) Answer D.

The primary purpose of annual audiometric testing is to monitor workers' hearing health as part of a comprehensive hearing conservation program. The OSHA requirements include provisions for insuring that the employees are provided hearing protection and given a baseline hearing test (audiogram). The noise reduction rating (NRR) of hearing protectors is compared to the sound level exposure for determining the appropriate attenuation. A sound level survey that demonstrates levels above 85 decibels requires a hearing conservation program. Supervisors are responsible for ensuring workers are trained and properly use PPE.

27)   Answer B.

There are several purposes and outcomes of safety meetings. The major purpose is to inform workers of job specific hazards.

28)   Answer C.

This is an essential tool of safety management for discovering and addressing the root causes of accidents. Applied behavior analysis helps the organization to assess the factors that are really driving its safety efforts. ABC analysis involves the following principles:

- Both antecedents (activators/triggers) and consequences influence behavior,
- Consequences influence behavior powerfully and directly, and
- Antecedents (activators, triggers) influence behavior indirectly, primarily serving to predict consequences.
  - The highest level of performance you can expect from the people you supervise is determined by the minimum standards you have established and maintained.
  - Actions influence performance: Remember that silence (failure to act) is consent.

This non-punitive approach characterizes the discussions and interviews with workers, developing a list of triggers or antecedents of the at-risk behavior. ABC Analysis has three fundamental steps:

1. Analyze the At-risk Behavior
2. Analyze the Safe Behavior
3. Draft the Action Plan

When a facility's safety effort is not working it is the consequences in favor of safe behavior are weaker than the consequences in favor of at-risk behavior.

There are three features that determine which consequences are stronger than others. The strongest behavioral consequences that are "soon, certain, and positive".

- **Timing.** A consequence that follows soon after a behavior influences behavior more effectively than consequences that occurs later. Again, silence is consent, thus failing to correct the unsafe act or at-risk behavior gives employees the indication that their behavior is acceptable and the behavior goes uncorrected. This may set precedence for continued at risk behaviors. In an effective safety program, the at-risk behavior is identified and corrected immediately and effectively through immediate resolution of the triggers.

- **Consistency.** A consequence that is certain to follow a behavior influences behavior more powerfully than an unpredictable or uncertain consequence. Failure to respond to each at risk behavior or failure to consistently reinforce the standard of performance will send mixed signals to employees. Prompt, consistent, and persistent corrective action is required. In any safety cultural change implementation, it is essential that all members of the team be informed of the consequence for at risk behavior, and that supervision enforces the rules. This lays the groundwork for predictable consequence.

- **Significance.** A positive consequence influences behavior more powerfully than a negative consequence. Punitive verses resolution: Resolution comes in the form of discussion, investigation of the behavior, in search of the underlying causes or antecedents that may have given the employee the misguided perception that has created the at-risk behavior. By talking with the employee and altering the perception, we have educated the employee without punitive action and have gained by-in for safe behavior.

Many safety programs are oriented toward penalties and punishments, rather like the traffic citation for speeding. The usual effect is not to change behavior, but rather to teach people not to get caught. Negative consequences are less powerful in their impact on worker behavior than positive consequences are. (Krause, 1997)

29)   Answer B.

An aerial lift is any vehicle-mounted device Used to elevate personnel, including:

- Extendable boom platforms,
- Aerial ladders,
- Articulating (jointed) boom platforms,
- Vertical towers,

Scissor lifts and aerial are mobile supported scaffold work platforms used to safely move workers vertically and to different locations in a variety of industries including construction, retail, entertainment and manufacturing. Scissor lifts are different from aerial lifts because the lifting mechanism moves the work platform straight up and down using crossed beams functioning in a scissor-like fashion. Although scissor lifts present hazards similar to scaffolding when extended and stationary, using scissor lifts safely depends on considering equipment capabilities, limitations and safe practices.

30)   Answer A.

The attachment of the body harness must be in the center of the wearer's back, near the shoulder level, or above the head. The components of fall protection system include an anchor, connection (lanyard) and body wear (harness). Body harnesses are designed to minimize stress forces on an employee's body in the event of a fall, while providing sufficient freedom of movement to allow work to be performed. Anchorages used for attachment of personal fall arrest equipment must be independent of any anchorage being used to support or suspend platforms, and capable of supporting at least 5,000 pounds per employee attached, or must be designed and used as follows:

- As part of a complete personal fall arrest system which maintains a safety factor of at least two.
- Under the supervision of a qualified person.

Vertical lifelines or lanyards must have a minimum breaking strength of 5,000 pounds, and be protected against being cut or abraded.

Each employee must be attached to a separate vertical lifeline, except during the construction of elevator shafts, where two employees may be attached to the same lifeline in the hoistway, provided:

- Both employees are working atop a false car that is equipped with guardrails.
- The strength of the lifeline is 10,000 pounds (5,000 pounds per employee).
- All other lifeline criteria have been met.

Self-retracting vertical lifelines and lanyards that automatically limit free fall distance to 2 feet or less must be capable of sustaining a minimum tensile load of 3,000 pounds when in the fully extended position. If they do not automatically limit the free fall to 2 feet or less, ripstitch lanyards, and tearing and deforming lanyards, must be capable of sustaining a minimum tensile load of 5,000 pounds when in the fully extended position

Horizontal lifelines are to be designed, installed, and used under the supervision of a qualified person, and as part of a complete personal fall arrest system which maintains a safety factor of at least two.

On suspended scaffolds or similar working platforms with horizontal lifelines that may become vertical lifelines, the devices used to connect to a horizontal lifeline must be capable of locking in both directions on the lifeline.

Connectors, including D-rings and snaphooks, must be made from drop-forged, pressed or formed steel, or equivalent materials. They must have a corrosion-resistant finish, with smooth surfaces and edges to prevent damage to connecting parts of the system.

D-Rings must have a minimum tensile strength of 5,000 pounds, and be proof-tested to a minimum tensile load of 3,600 pounds without cracking, breaking, or becoming permanently deformed.

Snaphooks must have a minimum tensile strength of 5,000 pounds, and be proof-tested to a minimum tensile load of 3,600 pounds without cracking, breaking, or becoming permanently deformed.

They must also be locking-type, double-locking, designed and used to prevent the disengagement of the snaphook by the contact of the snaphook keeper with the connected member. Unless it is designed for the following connections, snaphooks must not be engaged:

- Directly to webbing, rope, or wire.
- To each other.
- To a D-ring to which another snaphook or other connector is attached.
- To a horizontal lifeline.
- To any object which is incompatibly shaped in relation to the snaphook such that the connected object could depress the snaphook keeper and release itself.
- Ensure that personal fall arrest systems will, when stopping a fall:
  - Limit maximum arresting force to 1,800 pounds.
  - Be rigged such that an employee can neither free fall more than 6 feet nor contact any lower level.
  - Bring an employee to a complete stop and limit maximum deceleration distance to 3½ feet.
  - Have sufficient strength to withstand twice the potential impact energy of a worker free falling a distance of 6 feet, or the free fall distance permitted by the system, whichever is less
- Remove systems and components from service immediately if they have been subjected to fall impact, until inspected by a competent person and deemed undamaged and suitable for use.
- Promptly rescue employees in the event of a fall, or assure that they are able to rescue themselves.
- Inspect systems before each use for wear, damage, and other deterioration, and remove defective components from service.
- Do not attach fall arrest systems to guardrail systems or hoists.
- Rig fall arrest systems to allow movement of the worker only as far as the edge of the walking/working surface, when used at hoist areas

31)   Answer A.

Operator fatigue is an example of a human factor.

32) Answer A.

A safety procedure is an example of an administrative control which is part of the management system.

33) Answer C.

A sling at a 45-degree angle will reduce the SWL by 30%. A 45° angle is considered the minimum angle for rigging. The rated capacity of a sling varies depending upon the type of sling, the size of the sling, and the type of hitch. Operators must know the capacity of the sling. Charts or tables that contain this information generally are available from sling manufacturers. The values given are for new slings. Older slings must be used with additional caution. Under no circumstances shall a sling's rated capacity be exceeded. There are four primary factors to consider when safely lifting a load. They are (1) the size, weight, and center of gravity of the load; (2) the number of legs and the angle the sling makes with the horizontal line; (3) the rated capacity of the sling; and (4) the history of the care and usage of the sling.

34) Answer A.

Workers new to the job site must be trained initially and before exposed to the job site hazards.

35) Answer A.

All machines consist of three fundamental areas; the point of operation, the power transmission device, and the operating controls. Despite all machines having the same basic components, their safeguarding needs widely differ due to varying physical characteristics and operator involvement.

(OSHA, 2007) Machine Guarding eTool. *OSHA Machine Guarding eTool.*

36)   Answer D.

According to OSHA and NIOSH, effective heat stress management may include:

- Training for supervisors and workers to prevent, recognize, and treat heat-related illness
- Implementing a heat acclimatization program for workers,,
- Providing for and encouraging proper hydration with proper amounts and types of fluids
- Establishing work/rest schedules appropriate for the current heat stress conditions (an industrial hygienist may need to be consulted)
- Ensuring access to shade or cool areas
- Monitoring workers during hot conditions
- Providing prompt medical attention to workers who show signs of heat-related illness
- Evaluating work practices continually to reduce exertion and environmental heat stress
- Monitoring weather reports daily and rescheduling jobs with high heat exposure to cooler times of the day
- Workers should do the following:
- Drink water or other liquids frequently enough to never become thirsty (about 1 cup every 15–20 minutes). Hydration is the most important tool in preventing heat-related illness, and workers should try to be well-hydrated before arriving at work.
- Eat during lunch and other rest breaks. Food helps replace lost electrolytes.
- Wear light-colored, loose-fitting, breathable clothing such as cotton.
- Wear a wide-brimmed hat when possible.
- Take breaks in the shade or a cool area when possible.
- Be aware that protective clothing or personal protective equipment may increase the risk of heat stress.
- Monitor their physical condition and that of coworkers.
- Tell their supervisor if they have symptoms of heat-related illness.
- Talk with their doctor about medications they are taking and how the medications may affect their tolerance of heat.

NIOSH Criteria for a Recommended Standard Occupational Exposure to Heat and Hot Environments.

37)   Answer B.

When portable ladders are used for access to an upper landing surface, the ladder side rails shall extend at least 3 feet (0.9 m) above the upper landing surface to which the ladder is used to gain access; **or, when such an extension is not possible because of the ladder's length, then the ladder shall be secured at its top to a rigid support that will not deflect**, and a grasping device, such as a grab rail, shall be provided to assist employees in mounting and dismounting the ladder. In no case shall the extension be such that ladder deflection under a load would, by itself, cause the ladder to slip off its support.

38)   Answer B.

Carpal tunnel syndrome is defined as an injury or inflammation of the carpal tunnel located in the wrist. This injury is common among repetitive motion workers. The median nerve is compressed resulting in numbness, tingling and sometimes pain in the fingers and wrist.

Examples of Musculoskeletal Disorders				
Body Parts Affected	Symptoms	Possible Causes	Workers Affected	Disease Name
thumbs	pain at the base of the thumbs	twisting and gripping	butchers, housekeepers, packers, seamstresses, cutters	De Quervain's disease
fingers	difficulty moving finger; snapping and jerking movements	repeatedly using the index fingers	meatpackers, poultry workers, carpenters, electronic assemblers	trigger finger

shoulders	pain, stiffness	working with the hands above the head	power press operators, welders, painters, assembly line workers	rotator cuff tendinitis
hands, wrists	pain, swelling	repetitive or forceful hand and wrist motions	core making, poultry processing, meatpacking	tenosynovitis
fingers, hands	numbness, tingling; ashen skin; loss of feeling and control	exposure to vibration	chain saw, pneumatic hammer, and gasoline powered tool operators	Raynaud's syndrome (white finger)
fingers, wrists	tingling, numbness, severe pain; loss of strength, sensation in the thumbs, index, or middle or half of the ring fingers	repetitive and forceful manual tasks without time to recover	meat and poultry and garment workers, upholsterers, assemblers, VDT operators, cashiers	carpal tunnel syndrome
back	low back pain, shooting pain or numbness in the upper legs	whole body vibration	truck and bus drivers, tractor and subway operators; warehouse workers; nurses aides; grocery cashiers; baggage handlers	back disability

39)   Answer B.

The most important information on an SDS includes emergency procedures and first aid for chemical exposure.

40)   Answer D.

Anthropometry refers to the measurement of the human individual. Anthropometry involves the systematic measurement of the physical properties of the human body, primarily dimensional descriptors of body size and shape. Today, anthropometry plays an important role in industrial design, clothing design, ergonomics and architecture where statistical data about the distribution of body dimensions in the population are used to optimize products. Changes in lifestyles, nutrition, and ethnic composition of populations lead to changes in the distribution of body dimensions (e.g. the obesity epidemic) and require regular updating of anthropometric data collections.

Kinesiology is a scientific study of human or non-human body movement. Kinesiology addresses physiological, biomechanical, and psychological mechanisms of movement. Applications of kinesiology to human health (i.e. **human Kinesiology**) include biomechanics and orthopedics; strength and conditioning; sport psychology; methods of rehabilitation, such as physical and occupational therapy; and sport and exercise. Studies of human and animal motion include measures from motion tracking systems, electrophysiology of muscle and brain activity, various methods for monitoring physiological function, and other behavioral and cognitive research techniques.

Physiology is the scientific study of the normal function in living systems. A sub-discipline of biology, its focus is in how organisms, organ systems, organs, cells, and biomolecules carry out the chemical or physical functions that exist in a living system

Ergonomics (Human Factors) also known as comfort design, functional design, and systems, is the practice of designing products, systems, or processes to take proper account of the interaction between them and the people who use them. The study of people's efficiency in their working environment. The field has seen contributions from numerous disciplines, such as psychology, engineering, biomechanics, industrial design, physiology, and anthropometry. In essence, it is the study of designing equipment, devices and processes that fit the human body and its cognitive abilities. The two terms "human factors" and "ergonomics" are essentially synonymous.

41)   Answer C.

Irritants are chemicals that will irritate various tissues causing redness, rashes, swelling, coughing, or even hemorrhaging. Chlorine and ammonia are two examples of irritants.

Another name for **sensitizers** is allergens. These chemicals cause an allergic type of reaction due to sensitivity from prior exposure. An acute response may be swelling of the breathing tubes, which causes breathing difficulty. Sensitizers can cause chronic lung disease. Some common examples are epoxies, aromatic amines, formaldehyde, nickel metal, and maleic anhydride.

Mutagens cause alterations in the genes of an exposed person. The result may be malfunction of a specific organ or tissue, depending upon the type of cell in which the mutation took place. Gene damage can be passed on to children if the mutation occurred in either parent's sperm or egg. Examples of mutagens are ethylene oxide, benzene, and hydrazine.

Teratogens cause damage or death to a developing fetus. This damage cannot be passed on to further generations, as it does not affect the genetic code. Examples of teratogens are thalidomide, dioxins, lead, and cadmium.

42)   Answer A.

To determine the proper respirator, the chemical hazards must be known first. Next, consider the respirator assigned protection factor (APF), chemical concentrations in the workplace, and then the maximum use concentration (MUC). NIOSH definition Immediately Dangerous to Life or Health concentrations represent the maximum concentration from which, in the event of a respirator failure, one could escape within 30 minutes without a respirator and without experiencing any escape-impairing (e.g., severe eye irritation) or irreversible health effects.   An SCBA has the highest Assigned Protection Factor (APF). The APF means the workplace level of respiratory protection that a respirator or class of respirators is expected to provide to employees when the employer implements a continuing, effective respiratory protection program as specified by this section.

Assigned Protection Factors					
Type of Respirator	Quarter mask	Half mask	Full facepiece	Helmet/Hood	Loose-fitting
Air-Purifying Respirator	5	10	50	—	—
Powered Air-Purifying Respirator (PAPR)	—	50	1,000	25/1,000	25
Supplied-Air Respirator (SAR) or Airline Respirator				— 25/1,000	— 25
• Demand mode	—	10	50		
• Continuous flow mode	—	50	1,000	—	—
• Pressure-demand or other positive-pressure mode	—	50	1,000		
Self-Contained Breathing Apparatus (SCBA)					
• Demand mode	—	10	50	50	—
• Pressure-demand or other positive- pressure mode (e.g., open/closed circuit)—	—	—	10,000	10,000	—

OSHA 3352-02   2009   Assigned Protection Factors for the Revised Respiratory Protection Standard.

End-of-service-life indicator (ESLI) means a system that warns the respirator user of the approach of the end of adequate respiratory protection, for example, that the sorbent is approaching saturation or is no longer effective.

43)   Answer D.

The point of operation is the area on a machine where work is performed.

44)   Answer C.

Workers shall wear hard hats where there is a potential for objects falling from above, bumps to their heads from fixed objects, or accidental head contact with electrical hazards.

- Hard hats are routinely inspected for dents, cracks or deterioration.
- Hard hats are replaced after a heavy blow or electrical shock.
- Hard hats are maintained in good condition.

45)   Answer B.

All answer choices are important, but the most important action **before** beginning crane operations, is to check for overhead power lines.

46)   Answer B.

1926.1427(a) The employer must ensure that, prior to operating any equipment covered under subpart CC, the person is operating the equipment during a training period in accordance with paragraph (f) of this section, or the operator is qualified or certified to operate the equipment in accordance with the standard.

1926.602(c)(1)(vi) Lifting and hauling equipment (other than equipment covered under Subpart N of this part). (1)(vi) All industrial trucks in use shall meet the applicable requirements of design, construction, stability, inspection, testing, maintenance, and operation, as defined in American National Standards Institute B56.1-1969, *Safety Standards for Powered Industrial Trucks*. From ANSI Standard B56.1-1969, "Operator Training. Only trained and authorized operators shall be permitted to operate a powered industrial truck. Methods shall be devised to train operators in the safe operation of powered industrial trucks. Badges or other visual indication of the operators' authorization should be displayed at all times during work period."

47)   Answer D.

Do not overload. Know the stated capacity of your crane and do not exceed it. Only by keeping within the weight limit can you operate the crane safely.

48)   Answer B.

1926.251(a)(1) Rigging equipment for material handling shall be inspected prior to use on each shift and as necessary during its use to ensure that it is safe.

49)   Answer A.

For experienced workers, the most important task for a supervisor is to enforce safety rules on the job. The best course of action is to stop the work, correct the worker, and follow company disciplinary procedures.

50)   Answer A.

For inexperienced workers, the most important task for a supervisor is to ensure they know potential job hazards and how to protect themselves. The best course of action is to stop the work and educate the worker on job safety.

51)   Answer B.

Workers are more likely to follow rules when the supervisor leads by example and follow the rules.

52)   Answer D.

The term "**Universal Precautions,**" refers to a concept of bloodborne disease control, which requires that **all human blood and body fluids are treated as if known to be infectious** for HIV, HBV, and other bloodborne pathogens. Universal Precautions are not limited to PPE, but also include sharps management and contaminated equipment management procedures.

Bloodborne pathogens are infectious microorganisms in human blood that can cause disease in humans. These pathogens include, but are not limited to, hepatitis B (HBV), hepatitis C (HCV) and human immunodeficiency virus (HIV). Needle sticks and other sharps-related injuries may expose workers to bloodborne pathogens. These should be considered "contaminated sharps" and be disposed of properly in appropriate **sharps containers.** Workers in many occupations, including first responders, housekeeping personnel in some industries, nurses and other healthcare personnel, all may be at risk for exposure to bloodborne pathogens. In order to reduce or eliminate the hazards of occupational exposure to bloodborne pathogens, an employer must implement an **exposure control plan** for the worksite with details on employee protection measures. The plan must also describe how an employer will use engineering and work practice controls, personal protective clothing and equipment, employee training, medical surveillance, **hepatitis B vaccinations**, and other provisions as required by OSHA's Bloodborne Pathogens Standard (29 CFR 1910.1030).

53)   Answer B.

The assured equipment grounding conductor program covers all cord sets, receptacles which are not a part of the permanent wiring of the building or structure, and equipment connected by cord and plug which are available for use or used by employees. The requirements which the program must meet are stated in 29 CFR 1926.404(b)(1)(iii), but employers may provide additional tests or procedures. (See appendix.) OSHA requires that a written description of the employer's assured equipment grounding conductor program, including the specific procedures adopted, be kept at the jobsite. This program should outline the employer's specific procedures for required equipment inspections, tests, and test schedule. The required tests must be recorded, and the record maintained until replaced by a more current record. The written program description and recorded tests must be made available, at the jobsite, to OSHA and to any affected employee upon request. The employer is required to designate one or more **competent persons** to implement the program. Electrical equipment noted in the assured equipment grounding conductor program must be visually inspected for damage or defects before each day's use. Any damaged or defective equipment must **not** be used by the employee until repaired. Two tests are required by OSHA. One is a continuity test to ensure that the equipment grounding conductor is electrically continuous. It must be performed on all cord sets, receptacles which are not part of the permanent wiring of the building or structure, and on cord- and plug-connected equipment which is required to be grounded. This test may be performed using a simple continuity tester, such as a lamp and battery, a bell and battery, an ohmmeter, or a receptacle tester. The other test must be performed on receptacles and plugs to ensure that the equipment grounding conductor is connected to its proper terminal. This test can be performed with the same equipment used in the first test. These tests are required before first use, after any repairs, after damage is suspected to have occurred, and at 3-month intervals. Cord sets and receptacles which are essentially fixed and not exposed to damage must be tested at regular intervals not to exceed 6 months. Any equipment which fails to pass the required tests shall not be made available or used by employees.

54) Answer A.

Hazard: Any real or potential condition that can cause injury, illness, or death to personnel; damage to or loss of a system, equipment, or property; or damage to the environment. A potentially unsafe condition resulting from failures, malfunctions, external events, errors, or a combination thereof. A condition, set of circumstances or inherent property that can cause injury, illness or death.

Risk is defined as the combination of the severity of a defined exposure with its frequency of occurrence. The technique that effectively decreases a project's schedule risk without increasing the overall risk is to incorporate slack time into the project's critical path schedule early in project planning.

Probability: The likelihood of a hazard causing an incident or exposure that could result in harm or damage for a selected unit of time, events, population, items or activities being considered.

Severity: The extent of harm or damage that could result from a hazard related incident or exposures.

Risk analysis is the process of identifying safety risk. This involves identifying hazards that present mishap risk with an assessment of the risk.

Risk assessment is the process of determining the risk presented by the identified hazards. This involves evaluating the identified hazard causal factors and then characterizing the risk as the product of the hazard severity times the hazard probability.

55)   Answer B.

Risk is defined as the probability that a substance or situation will produce harm under specified conditions. Risk is a combination of two factors:

1) The probability that an adverse event will occur and

2) The consequences of the adverse event.

Risk encompasses impacts on public health and environment, and arises from exposure and hazard. Risk does not exist if exposure to a harmful substance or situation does not or will not occur. Hazard is determined by whether a particular substance or situation has the potential to cause harmful effects. Risk is the probability of a specific outcome, generally adverse, given a particular set of conditions.

56)   Answer B.

Hazard elimination is the best solution.

57)   Answer C.

A loss control system must be able to identify the hazardous conditions as well as understand the real risks associated with those hazardous conditions. A loss control system is incomplete if it solely identifies hazardous conditions and does not act to understand the risks. Therefore, the actions taken are relative to the risks associated with the hazardous conditions.

58)   Answer B.

Aerosol - Suspension of fine liquid or solid particles dispersed in air.

Mist - Suspension of liquid particles in air formed by condensation from vapor or by some mechanical process ($40 - 400\mu m$).

Fume - Solid particle aerosol formed by condensation from the vapor state ($0.001 - 0.2\mu m$).

Smoke - aerosol formed from combustion of organic material ($0.01 - 0.5\mu m$).

Dust - Particulate material generated by a mechanical process ($0.5 - 50\ \mu m$).

59)   Answer D.

According to OSHA publication 3074 hearing Conservation, Employers must provide at least two types of hearing protection and instruct employees on proper use/wearing. Employers must provide employees with a selection of at least one variety of hearing plug and one variety of hearing muff. OSHA 1910.95 & 1926.52 occupational noise. 1926.101(b) Ear protective devices inserted in the ear shall be fitted or determined individually by competent persons.

60)   Answer A.

Securing the area is critically important for evidence preservation.

61)   Answer B.

Authorized workers must know the specific energy isolation locations and devices for each individual piece of equipment.

62)   Answer B.

The Supervisor is considered the most influential person for worker safety. Enforcing the use of PPE is a common supervisory role in a safety management system.

63)   Answer A.

Develop a system for the general contractor and subcontractors to share the SDS.

64)   Answer A.

According to Haight (2012), there are four major phases of development in a system life cycle: (1) concept, (2) system development, (3) production and deployment, and (4) sustainment and disposal. Each phase includes safety engineering tasks that result in a formal decision about proceeding to the next phase. A system-safety management plan should be developed during the concept phase in order to design safety into the system and maintain it through-out the system's life. Incorporating system safety early in development increases the probability that hazards can be addressed more economically and with greater efficiency. A formal decision earmarks the acceptance of risks) to that point of development or operation.

65)   Answer C.

Fostering foreman and supervisor involvement is critical to an effective safety and health management system.

66)   Answer B.

Read and understand the hazards on the JSA and make any corrections to it prior to use. The revised version should be sent to the company safety officer.

67)   Answer A.

Interviewing witnesses separately is best practice for accident investigation.

68)   Answer B.

Studies indicate that the systematic positive reinforcement of appropriate behavior is highly effective with improving individual safety performance.

69)   Answer B.

According to the National Safety Council, the primary purpose of accident investigation is to prevent recurrence based on similar causes.

70)   Answer C.

Supervisor's attitude has a direct influence on the employee's safety performance.

71)   Answer A.

Safety training objectives must be aligned with on the job safe work objectives. Supervisors should ensure that safety training is specific and relevant to the job hazards and how a worker can protect oneself.

72)   Answer A.

Supervisors should continuously give positive reinforcement for good work practice and discuss hazards and corrective measures.

73)   Answer B.

According to the NSC Supervisors' Safety Manual, there are four distinct steps in the listening process.

- *Sensing.* The first step is purely mechanical: Did the listener hear the words that were spoken? If he or she can repeat the sense of the words, this step
  has taken place.
- *Interpreting.* How did the listener understand the words that were spoken? The same words can have different meanings for speaker and listener.
  Follow-up questions may be needed at this stage.
- *Evaluating.* At this stage, the listener determines whether he or she agrees with the message. Evaluation can take place only after the listener understands the message.
- *Responding.* Response may be a simple nod or shake of the head or an "I see." Before making a lengthier response, the listener should be sure the speaker has finished a point.

Most people speak at about 125 to 150 words per minute. Yet most people can listen at speeds of 600 or more words per minute. That time differential might seem to ensure good listening. In fact, many people have so much downtime while trying to listen that their minds wander. That is one reason why they hear and remember only 25% to 30% of what is said. Effective listeners use the time differential to think along with the speaker, mentally outlining the points.

They evaluate the speaker's credibility and analyze whether his or her nonverbal messages agree with the verbal ones. Making good use of the time differential can help people improve their understanding, the key to communications. Consider the following guidelines for improved effective listening:

- Stop talking. You can't listen while you are talking.
- Repeat/paraphrase. Once the speaker is finished, repeat what you heard to verify your understanding.

- Clarify/probe. If any of the message is unclear to you, ask questions until you understand it.
- Maintain eye contact. Meeting the speaker's eye helps you concentrate on what is being said. It also shows that you are paying attention.
- Empathize. Put yourself in the speaker's place to get a better understanding of why he or she holds the opinions expressed.
- Share responsibility for communication. The receiver is just as responsible as the sender for good communication.

There is also some don'ts to remember: Don't interrupt, don't make assumptions, and don't jump to conclusions (think before you respond).

74)   Answer D.

Hard hats are required when performing work in areas where: the possibility of falling objects exists; around energized electrical lines; where overhead hazards such as piping exist; around heavy equipment. Overhead hazards that are greater than 7 feet from the working surface are generally considered guarded by distance.

75)   Answer C.

Manufacturer's recommendations are the primary resource for operating tools and equipment.

76)   Answer A.

Back braces are not considered by OSHA to be a form of PPE.

77)   Answer A.

Chemical goggles and face shield provide the best eye and face protection from splashing while pouring chemicals.

78)   Answer D.

Motivation involves moving people to action that will support the company's desired goals. In occupational safety and health, motivation increases employees' awareness, interest, and willingness to act in ways that improve their own safety and that of co-workers.

Motivation aims primarily at changing behavior and attitudes. It is generally defined by three factors: (1) direction of behavior, (2) intensity of action, and

(3) persistence of effort.

Motivation efforts should support the mainline safety, health, and environmental system, not take its place. Chances of success increase when the following factors are present:

- Management demonstrates its commitment at every opportunity.
- The program is energized through performance recognition, and discipline.
- Workplace conditions are safe and healthful.
- Tools, equipment, and workplace layout are designed appropriately.
- Maintenance is effective.
- Training and supervision are effective.

79) Answer A.

Nausea, sweating, dizziness are symptoms of heat exhaustion.

80) Answer B.

The four major exposure paths for chemicals to enter into the body are:

- Inhalation
- Eye/skin contact (absorption)
- Ingestion
- Injection

81) Answer A.

Bloodborne pathogens standard requires that people must be trained when cleaning up human blood and body fluids

82)   Answer C.

Key definitions for energy isolation:

- Energy-isolating device: A mechanical device that physically prevents the transmission or release of energy, including but not limited to the following: A manually operated electrical circuit breaker; a disconnect switch; a manually operated switch by which the conductors of a circuit can be disconnected from all ungrounded supply conductors and, in addition, no pole can be operated independently; a line valve; a block; and any similar device used to block or isolate energy. Push buttons, selector switches and other control circuit type devices are not energy isolating devices.
- Authorized employee: An employee who locks or tags machines or equipment in order to perform servicing or maintenance.
- Affected employee: An employee who is required to use machines or equipment on which servicing is performed under the Lockout/Tagout standard or who performs other job responsibilities in an area where such servicing is performed.
- Other employees: All employees who are or may be in an area where energy control procedures may be utilized.
- Capable of being locked out: An energy-isolating device is considered capable of being locked out if it:
  - Is designed with a hasp or other means of attachment to which a lock can be affixed.
  - Has a locking mechanism built into it.
  - Can be locked without dismantling, rebuilding, or replacing the energy-isolating device or permanently altering its energy control capability.
- Energized: Machines and equipment are energized when they are connected to an energy source or they contain residual or stored energy.
- Energy source: Any source of electrical, mechanical, hydraulic, pneumatic, chemical, thermal, or other energy.
- Lockout: The placement of a lockout device on an energy-isolating device, in accordance with an established procedure, ensuring that the energy-isolating device and the equipment being controlled cannot be operated until the lockout device is removed.

- Lockout device: Any device that uses positive means, such as a lock, blank flanges and bolted slip blinds, to hold an energy-isolating device in a safe position, thereby preventing the energizing of machinery or equipment.
- Normal production operations: Utilization of a machine or equipment to perform its intended production function.
- Servicing and/or maintenance: Workplace activities such as constructing, installing, setting up, adjusting, inspecting, modifying, maintaining and/or servicing machines or equipment, including lubrication, cleaning or unjamming of machines or equipment, and making adjustments or tool changes, where employees could be exposed to the unexpected energization or startup of the equipment or release of hazardous energy.
- Tagout: The placement of a tagout device on an energy-isolating device, in accordance with an established procedure, to indicate that the energy-isolating device and the equipment being controlled may not be operated until the tagout device is removed.
- Tagout device: Any prominent warning device, such as a tag and a means of attachment, that can be securely fastened to an energy-isolating device to indicate that the machine or equipment to which it is attached may not be operated until the tagout device is removed.

83)   Answer A.

According to the National Safety Council accident investigation should be conducted to provide the facts, if fault-finding is attempted the investigation may cause more harm than good. Mishap investigation is conducted to determine both obvious and hidden cause factors. It does tend to serve as the baseline for further analysis, but *to determine the facts surrounding the event* is the primary reason for investigation.

84)   The best selection is answer D because

Every employer has a shared responsibility for safety at multiple-employee work sites.

85)   Answer B.

Valve protection caps must be secured when transporting, moving or storing compressed cylinders. OSHA 1926.350(a)(1)

86)   Answer B.

Emergency planning for an emergency should be done prior to work beginning at the site.

87)   Answer B.

The three primary types of emergency eyewash and shower stations include (ANSI Z358.1-2014):

- Eyewash stations for splashes or spills where only the eyes are likely affected—Require flushing of 0.4 gallons per minute at 30 PSI for **15 minutes**.
- Eye/face wash equipment for splashes or spills where the eyes *and* face are affected—Require flushing of 3.0 gallons per minute at 30 PSI for 15 minutes.
- Emergency showers for splashes or spills that affect the larger areas of the body—Require flushing of 20 gallons per minute at 30 PSI for 15 minutes.

Two different types of eyewash stations are acceptable under the ANSI Z 358.1 standard:

- Plumbed permanent eyewash stations
- Self-contained, gravity-fed portable shower and eyewash stations

Plumbed stations are permanently connected to a source of potable water, whereas portable stations are self-contained gravity-fed units with their own flushing fluid that must be replaced after each use. The ANSI Z358.1 standard states that the water temperature for the flushing fluid in an eyewash station **must be tepid,** which is between 60° and 100° F or 16° and 38° C. Tepid water helps encourage worker compliance to meet the full 15 minutes of flushing which helps prevent further absorption of chemicals and injury to the eyes. Eyewash stations should be located on the same level as the hazard in a well-lit area that is properly marked as an emergency eyewash station. It must be positioned within 10 seconds (about 55 feet) of the hazard along a path that is free of obstructions. An obstruction-free path is critical because the vision of injured workers is impaired. ANSI Z358.1 requires that plumbed flushing stations "be activated weekly for a period long enough to verify operation and ensure that flushing fluid is available." ANSI states that portable equipment "be **visually** checked to determine if flushing fluid needs to be changed or supplemented." Whether plumbed or portable, both types also need to be tested annually and maintained according to the manufacturer's guidelines. The OSHA requirements for emergency eyewashes and showers, found at 29 CFR 1910.151(c), specify that "where the eyes or body of any person may be exposed to injurious corrosive materials, suitable facilities for quick drenching or flushing of the eyes and body shall be provided within the work area for immediate emergency use. As the standard states, an eyewash and/or safety shower would be required where an employee's eyes or body could be exposed to injurious corrosive materials. If none of the materials used in this work area is an injurious corrosive [chemical] (as indicated by the Safety Data Sheet (SDS) for each product), then an emergency eyewash or shower would not be required pursuant to 1910.151(c).

88)   Answer C.

The investigation process should begin after arranging for first aid or medical treatment for the injured person(s). In getting started, remind everyone involved, especially workers, the investigation is to learn and prevent, not find fault. Steps of the investigation process include:

1. Call or gather the necessary person(s) to conduct the investigation and obtain the investigation kit.
2. Secure the area where the injury occurred and preserve the work area as it is.
3. Identify and gather witnesses to the injury event.
4. Interview the involved worker.
5. Interview all witnesses.
6. Document the scene of the injury through photos or videos.
7. Complete the investigation report, including determination of what caused the incident and what corrective actions will prevent recurrences.
8. Use results to improve the injury and illness prevention program to better identify and control hazards before they result in incidents.
9. Ensure follow-up on completion of corrective actions.

89)   Answer A.

At minimum, documentation of training includes, student name, topic outline, objectives, date, instructor name and qualifications.

90)   Answer A.

Research has shown that a positive environment encourages better safety by workers than an environment based strictly on enforcement. Enforcement is an important aspect of a safety program, but positive encouragement before enforcement is best. It is crucial to set a positive example as the supervisor by following **all** safety requirements. The supervisor needs to follow up on all complaints and hazard reports.

91)   The best selection is answer D because

Training is provided to impart knowledge and ability. In the case of safety training, the primary objective is to impart knowledge and ability to allow a worker to prevent injuries and accidents.

92)   Answer A.

Top management demonstration of commitment and support is critical for an effective safety management system.

93)   Answer A.

It is critical that the electricity source that caused the shock be secured to prevent self and others from being shocked while helping the victim. If the victim is still in contact with an energized electrical circuit, rescuers can be shocked when they touch the victim. (2009) NIOSH Publication No. 2009-113: *Electrical Safety: Safety*

94)   Answer C.

Take out of service, tag it, and inform crew not to use is the best solution.

95)   Answer C.

The ground wire is not necessary to complete the circuit with the electrical equipment load. Electrical equipment can be operated with the ground wire disconnected. An example of this would be when the third prong on a three-wire extension cord is missing.

96)   Answer B.

A check valve, pressure regulator, hydraulic seal, or combination of these devices shall be provided at each station outlet, including those on portable headers, to prevent backflow. Portable outlet headers for fuel-gas service shall be provided with an approved hydraulic back-pressure valve installed at the inlet and preceding the service outlets, unless an approved pressure-reducing regulator, an approved back-flow check valve, or an approved hydraulic back-pressure valve is installed at each outlet. Outlets provided on headers for oxygen service may be fitted for use with pressure-reducing regulators or for direct hose connection.

97)   Answer D.

According to the National Safety Council publication, *Basics of Safety and Health,* common methods of hazard control, in order of precedence, are: designing out the hazard, eliminating the hazard by substitution or automation, reducing exposure, and using personal protective equipment. The following hierarchy of controls are prioritized from most effective to least effective. **(Adapted from ANSI-Z10)**

CONTROLS	EXAMPLES
1. Elimination	Design to eliminate hazards: falls, HAZMAT, confined spaces, materials handling, tools and machinery, etc.
2. Substitution	Substitute for less hazardous materials and equipment, reduce energy, etc.
3. Engineering Controls	Incorporate safety trough design such as: Ventilation systems, enclosures, guarding, interlocks, lift tables, conveyors, etc.
4. Warnings	Strategically place signs, alarms, enunciators, labels, etc.
5. Administrative Controls	Standard Operating Procedures (SOPs) such as: Conduct JSAs, job rotation, inspections, training, mentoring, etc.
6. Personal Protective Equipment	PPE assessments may result in the use of: safety glasses, goggles, face shields, fall protection, protective footwear, gloves, respirators, chemical suits, etc.

98) Answer A.

According to OSHA and NIOSH, to understand the best way to set up a computer workstation, it is helpful to understand the concept of neutral body positioning. This is a comfortable working posture in which joints are naturally aligned. Working with the body in a neutral position reduces stress and strain on the muscles, tendons, and skeletal system and reduces risk of developing a musculoskeletal disorder (MSD). The following are important considerations when attempting to maintain neutral body postures while working at the computer workstation:

- *Hands*, *wrists*, and *forearms* are straight, in-line and roughly parallel to the floor.
- *Head* is level, or bent slightly forward, forward facing, and balanced. Generally it is in-line with the *torso*.
- *Shoulders* are relaxed and *upper arms* hang normally at the side of the body.
- *Elbows* stay in close to the body and are bent between 90 and 120 degrees.
- *Feet* are fully supported by the floor or a footrest may be used if the desk height is not adjustable.
- *Back* is fully supported with appropriate lumbar support when sitting vertical or leaning back slightly.
- *Thighs* and *hips* are supported by a well-padded seat and generally parallel to the floor.
- *Knees* are about the same height as the hips with the *feet* slightly forward.

Regardless of how good working posture is, working in the same posture or sitting still for prolonged periods is not healthy. Research has linked sitting for long periods of time with a number of health concerns, including obesity and metabolic syndrome, a cluster of conditions that includes increased blood pressure, high blood sugar, excess body fat around the waist and abnormal cholesterol levels. Too much sitting also seems to increase the risk of death from cardiovascular disease and cancer. The working position should be changed frequently throughout the day in the following ways:

- Make small adjustments to chair or backrest.
- Stretch the fingers, hands, arms, and torso.
- Stand up and walk around for a few minutes periodically

99)   Answer A.

Effective safety and health activities are incorporated into business operations and are integrated into already functioning activities, whenever possible. Many existing activities in a business are already safety-related. This is particularly true with maintenance activities, such as a periodic inspection of electrical equipment.

100)   Answer D.

Authorized employee: An employee who locks out or tags out machines or equipment in order to perform servicing or maintenance on that machine or equipment. An affected employee becomes an authorized employee when that employee's duties include performing servicing or maintenance covered under this section.

Affected employee: An employee whose job requires him or her to operate or use a machine or equipment on which servicing, or maintenance is being performed under lockout or tagout, or whose job requires him or her to work in an area in which such servicing or maintenance is being performed.

Attendant: An employee assigned to remain immediately outside the entrance to an enclosed or other space to render assistance as needed to employees inside the space.

References

These published references provide reasonable coverage on the subject matter associated with the STSC Examination Blueprint and used in the content of this workbook. Examination items are not necessarily taken directly from these sources. Similar references also present acceptable coverage on the subject matter.

1). Aronsson, Gunnar (1999). Contingent Workers and Health and Safety, Work Employment & Society, *13* (3).

2). Board of Certified Safety Professionals (2013). BCSP Code of Ethics Retrieved 3/15/2016 from http://www.bcsp.org/Portals/0/Assets/DocumentLibrary/BCSPcodeofethics.pdf

3). Board of Certified Safety Professionals (2016). Complete Guide to the STS and STSC Application and Examination Information Retrieved 3/15/2016 from http://www.bcsp.org/Portals/0/Assets/DocumentLibrary/STS-STSC-Complete-Guide.pdf

4). Brauer, Roger (2006), Safety and Health for Engineers 2nd ed. Hoboken: John Wiley & Sons.

5). Bust, Phillip D. (Ed.) (2009), Contemporary Ergonomics 2009: Proceedings of the International Conference on Contemporary Ergonomics 2009 1st ed. Abingdon: Taylor & Francis.

6). Cantonwine, Sheila Cullen (1999). Safety Training That Delivers: How to Design and Present Better Technical Training Park Ridge: American Society of Safety Engineers.

7). Center for Process Safety (1992), Guidelines for Hazard Evaluation Procedures 2nd ed. New York: American Institute of Chemical Engineers.

8). Cote, Arthur; Bugbee, Percy (1991). Principles of Fire Protection Quincy: National Fire Protection Association.

9). Dainty, Andrew; Loosemore, Martin (Ed.) (2012) Human Resource Management in Construction: Critical Perspectives. London:

Routledge.

10). DiBerardinis, Louis (1999), Handbook of Occupational Safety and Health 2nd ed. Hoboken: John Wiley & Sons.

11). Ellis, J. Nigel (2011), Introduction to Fall Protection 4th ed. Park Ridge: American Society of Safety Engineers.

12). Gagnet, Grace Drennan (2000), Fall Protection and Scaffolding Safety 1st ed. Lanham: Government Institutes, Scarecrow Press.

13). Grote, Dick (1995), Discipline Without Punishment: The Proven Strategy That Turns Problem Employees Into Superior Performers 1st ed. New York: AMACOM.

14). Hagan, Phillip E.; Montgomery, John F.; O'Reilly, James T. (2009), Accident Prevention Manual for Business and Industry: Administration and Programs 13th ed. Itasca: National Safety Council.

15). Hagan, Phillip E.; Montgomery, John F.; O'Reilly, James T. (2009), Accident Prevention Manual for Business and Industry: Engineering and Technology 13th ed. Itasca: National Safety Council.

16). Haight, Joel (Ed.) (2008). The Safety Professional's Handbook: Technical Applications Park Ridge: American Society of Safety Engineers.

17). Hill, Daryl (2004), Construction Safety Management and Engineering 1st ed. Park Ridge: American Society of Safety Engineers.

18). International Association of Electrical Inspectors (2008), Soares Book on Grounding and Bonding 10th ed. Richardson: International Association of Electrical Inspectors.

19). Kelley, Stephen M. (2001). Lockout Tagout: A Practical Approach Park Ridge: American Society of Safety Engineers.

20). Krause, Thomas R. (1997), The Behavior-Based Safety Process: Managing Involvement for an Injury-Free Culture 2nd ed. New York: Van Nostrand Reinhold.

21). Krieger, Gary (2000), Accident Prevention Manual for Business and Industry: Environmental Management 2nd ed. Itasca: National Safety Council.

22). Ladou, Joseph (2007), Current Occupational and Environmental Medicine 4th ed. New York: McGraw-Hill Medical.

23). Levy, Barry S.; Wegman, David H.; Baron, Sherry L.; Sokas, Rosemary K. (2010). Occupational and Environmental Health: Recognizing and Preventing Disease and Injury Oxford: Oxford University Press.

24). MacCollum, David (1995), Construction Safety Planning, 1st ed. Hoboken: John Wiley & Sons.

25). MacDonald, Joseph A.; Rossnagel, W.; Higgins, Lindley (2009), Handbook of Rigging: Lifting, Hoisting, and Scaffolding for Construction and Industrial Operations 5th ed. New York: McGraw-Hill.

26). McManus, Neil (1999). Safety and Health in Confined Spaces Boca Raton: CRC Press.

27). National Fire Protection Association (2004), NFPA 70E: Handbook for Electrical Safety in the Workplace 1st ed. Clifton: Delmar Cengage Learning.

28). National Safety Council (2008), Supervisor's Safety Manual 10th ed. Itasca: National Safety Council.

29). Occupational Safety and Health Administration (2011). OSHA: Protecting Yourself from Noise in Construction Retrieved 3/15/2016 from https://www.osha.gov/Publications/3498noise-in-construction-pocket-guide.pdf

30). Petersen, Dan (2001), Safety Management: A Human Approach 3rd ed. Park Ridge: American Society of Safety Engineers.

31). Peterson, Dan (1999), Safety Supervision 2nd ed. Park Ridge: American Society of Safety Engineers.

32). Peyton, Robert X., Rubio, Toni C. (1991), Construction Safety Practices and Principles 1st ed. New York: Van Nostrand Reinhold.

33). Plog, Barbara A.; Quinlan, Patricia J. (2012), Fundamentals of Industrial Hygiene 6th ed. Itasca: National Safety Council.

34). Scott, Ronald (1997), Basic Concepts of Industrial Hygiene 1st ed. Boca Raton: CRC Press.

35). Snyder, Daniel J. (2014), Pocket Guide to Safety Essentials, 2nd ed. Itasca: National Safety Council.

36). Snyder, Daniel, J. (2013), Hazardous Materials Management Desk Reference 3rd ed. Bethesda Maryland: Alliance of Hazardous Materials Professionals

37). Swartz, George (1999), Forklift Safety: A Practical Guide to Preventing Powered Industrial Truck Incidents and Injuries 1st ed. Lanham: Government Institutes, Scarecrow Press.

38). Swartz, George, (Ed.) (2000). Safety Culture and Effective Safety Management Itasca: National Safety Council.

39). Sweet, Justin; Schneier, Marc (2012). Legal Aspects of Architecture, Engineering and the Construction Process Stamford: Cengage Learning.

40). Turner, Joe M. (2009), Excavation Systems: Planning, Design, and Safety 1st ed. New York: McGraw-Hill.

41). Weinstein, Michael B. (1997). Total Quality Safety Management and Auditing Boca Raton: CRC Press.

42). Weiss, W.H. (1982), Supervisor's Standard Reference Handbook 1st ed. Englewood Cliffs: Prentice-Hall Inc.

43). Yates, D. W. (2011). *Safety Professional's Reference and Study Guide* . Park Ridge: American Society of Safety Engineers.